A Study Guide
to accompany
THE HUMAN BRAIN

John Nolte, Ph.D.
Professor of Anatomy
Director, Division of Academic Resources
The University of Arizona College of Medicine
Tucson, Arizona

With 102 illustrations

Mosby-Year Book
ST. LOUIS   WASHINGTON, D.C.   TORONTO
1993

Editor: *Robert Farrell*
Design: *Jack Nolte*

Cover: Reproduction of a drawing by Rene Descartes in *De Homine*, 1662. Descartes thought that the pineal gland was the seat of the soul, monitoring the movement of "animal spirits" in sensory nerves and controlling the movement of animal spirits through motor nerves.

International Standard Book Number 0-8016-6332-6

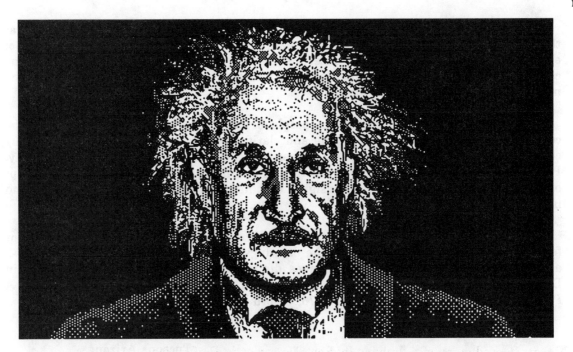

"Everything should be made as simple as possible, but not simpler."
-Albert Einstein

PREFACE

This is a book for students. Specifically, it is a book for students trying to review neuroanatomy or to distill out the important facts and concepts of human neuroanatomy. I tried to make it an account that would be useful by itself, so it does not depend too much on *The Human Brain* (C.V. Mosby Co., third edition, 1993) to make sense. However, it does parallel *The Human Brain* in its organization and should be particularly useful when used in conjunction with that book. In order to keep this *Study Guide* brief some background material was omitted, so it may not be productive to read the book with no prior knowledge of the subject. At the end of each chapter is a list of a few questions dealing specifically with the learning objectives for that chapter. The last chapter is a longer list of questions that often cover multiple topics. Whenever the answer to a question is not a simple definition or fact, a brief explanation is included. The clinical questions are fictions that are meant to illustrate neuroanatomical concepts. They are not intended to be clinically accurate or to make light of neurological disease. There are references here and there to figures in this *Study Guide* and also to figures in the second edition of *The Human Brain*. In order to differentiate between them, figures in *The Human Brain* are referred to as "text Fig.__."

I wanted to call this book *Translucent Neuroanatomy* (the publisher wouldn't let me), in the hope that it makes a difficult subject almost clear. What I tried to do is list and explain succinctly the really crucial material in *The Human Brain*. I did it mainly by compiling and adapting the list of learning objectives dealing with neuroanatomical topics that we use in the course I teach in at The University of Arizona College of Medicine. My list is unlikely to coincide exactly with that used by others, but it should overlap substantially.

My hope is that the lists of learning objectives define the core material clearly, that the text explains this material lucidly, and that the questions and explanations at the end of each chapter will allow you to determine your level of understanding with some confidence. I welcome comments on content or format, from students or faculty, so that the next version can be nearly transparent.

As always, I owe thanks to many people for their help. Students who have taken the course in years past have helped hone and clarify the learning objectives. My teaching colleagues, especially Pam Eller, Tom Finger and Steve Ringel helped in a similar way. Pam Eller, Meg Bradley, Monica Cooper-Abarca and Robert Gibbons read the manuscript of an earlier edition and provided insights that had evaded me. Carol was patient and urged me on.

Some of the figures include clip art from Wetpaint® (Dubl-Click Software, Inc.) or from ClickArt® (T/Maker Company); the drawings of a cerebral hemisphere in Fig. 15-1 and similar figures are based on images digitized and simplified from drawings in DeArmond, S. J., Fusco, M. M. and Dewey, M.M.: *Structure of the Human Brain, A Photographic Atlas*, ed. 2, New York, 1976, Oxford University Press.

John Nolte
Tucson, Arizona
September 1992

A STUDY GUIDE TO ACCOMPANY
THE HUMAN BRAIN

CONTENTS

viii

ILLUSTRATIONS

CHAPTER 1A

GENERAL ORGANIZATION OF THE CENTRAL NERVOUS SYSTEM

LEARNING OBJECTIVES

1. With respect to the nervous system, define each of the following terms: white matter, gray matter, nucleus, ganglion, cortex, tract. In cases where a tract has a two-part name, indicate the meaning of the first and second part. Indicate whether each of the following terms refers to a collection of neuronal cell bodies or a collection of axons: fasciculus, lemniscus, peduncle.

2. List the major subdivisions of the central nervous system, and the principal components of each of these subdivisions. In general terms, describe the functions of each of these components (e.g., Where are the basal ganglia and what are they involved with? What's a brainstem for?)

3. Define primary afferent neuron (vs. second- or higher-order), and indicate the location of the cell bodies of primary afferent neurons and the side of nervous system on which their central processes terminate. Similarly, define lower motor neuron, and indicate the location of the cell bodies of lower motor neurons and the side of the body in which their peripheral processes terminate.

4. Diagram the typical distribution pattern of somatosensory information within the central nervous system, indicating the points at which information crosses the midline and explaining why damage to sensory areas of the cerebral cortex typically causes contralateral deficits. Indicate the ways in which the distribution patterns of other types of sensory information may differ from the somatosensory pattern.

5. Diagram the general pattern of the corticospinal, basal ganglia and cerebellar systems, indicating the points at which information crosses the midline. Using this diagram, explain why damage to the corticospinal system often causes deficits contralateral to the lesion, damage to the basal ganglia system always causes deficits contralateral to the lesion, and damage to the cerebellar system usually causes deficits ipsilateral to the lesion. Explain why damage to any of these systems causes little or no sensory deficit.

The brain seems bewilderingly complex the first few times you look at it. One way to ease the bewilderment is to have an overview of some vocabulary and organizing principles, which Chapters 1A and 2 attempt to provide.

This first chapter goes a little beyond the contents of Chapter 1 in *The Human Brain*. It assumes you know a bit about the cellular organization of neurons and glial cells, then reviews some terminology and discusses the major ways in which big chunks of the central nervous system are wired together.

1. Neuronal cell bodies and axons are largely segregated from each other in the central nervous system.

The central nervous system (CNS) is separated to a great extent into areas of gray matter, containing neuronal cell bodies and dendrites, and areas of white matter, containing axons. Since most synapses are made onto neuronal cell bodies and dendrites, gray matter contains the sites of neural information processing and white matter is like telephone cables interconnecting these sites.

A specific area of gray matter is often referred to as a nucleus (e.g., trigeminal motor nucleus); when it forms a surface covering, it may be referred to as a cortex (e.g., cerebral cortex, cerebellar cortex). Ganglion usually refers to a group of neuronal cell bodies in the peripheral nervous system, but is also used occasionally to refer to masses of CNS gray matter (e.g., basal ganglia).

Specific groups of fibers in areas of white matter are often called tracts, and usually have two-part names that indicate the origin and termination of the fibers. For example, the corticospinal tract consists of axons that originate from cells in the cerebral cortex and terminate in the spinal cord. Several other terms are used to refer to structurally prominent areas of white matter; the most common are fasciculus, lemniscus and peduncle.

2. The central nervous system is composed of the cerebral hemispheres, diencephalon, brainstem, cerebellum and spinal cord.

The central nervous system is made up of the brain and the spinal cord. The brain in turn is composed of the cerebrum (forebrain), cerebellum and brainstem. The cerebrum, by far the largest component, is itself composed of the cerebral hemispheres and the diencephalon (from a Greek word meaning "in-between-brain" because it is interposed between the cerebral hemispheres and the brainstem).

Each cerebral hemisphere has a covering of cerebral cortex and encloses a series of large nuclei. Some of the enclosed nuclei (lenticular and caudate nuclei) are members of the basal ganglia, which help control movement; another (the amygdala) is part of the limbic system, which deals with drives and emotions. The cerebral cortex is a critical structure for perception, for the initiation of voluntary movement, and for the functions we think of as distinctively human—things like language and reasoning. Corresponding to these several functions, there are cortical areas primarily concerned with sensation, others with movement, and still others with more complex activities. Because of this parceling of functions, it is possible for cortical damage to impair some abilities while leaving others more or less unaffected.

The diencephalon includes the thalamus, a relay station for information on its way to the cerebral cortex, and the hypothalamus, which controls the autonomic nervous system and many aspects of drive-related behavior. The brainstem is subdivided into the medulla, pons and midbrain. It contains most of the cranial nerve nuclei, as well as long tracts on their way to or from the forebrain. The cerebellum is interconnected with most other parts of the CNS and, like the basal ganglia, helps control movement.

Major Division	Subdivisions	Principal Function
Cerebral hemisphere	cerebral cortex	cognition, memory, voluntary movement
	lenticular nucleus	part of basal ganglia: movement control
	caudate nucleus	part of basal ganglia: movement control
	amygdala	part of limbic system: drives and emotions
Diencephalon	thalamus	relays information to cerebral cortex
	hypothalamus	controls autonomic nervous system
Brainstem	medulla	cranial nerve nuclei; long tracts
	pons	cranial nerve nuclei; long tracts
	midbrain	cranial nerve nuclei; long tracts
Cerebellum		coordination of movement

3. Sensory neurons have cell bodies in the periphery and central processes that do not cross the midline. Motor neurons have cell bodies in the central nervous system and axons that do not cross the midline.

The CNS communicates with the rest of the body primarily through sensory neurons and motor neurons. Primary sensory neurons either have specialized, receptive endings outside the CNS or have peripheral endings that receive connections from separate receptor cells. Primary sensory neurons typically have their cell bodies in ganglia adjacent to the CNS, and central processes that synapse in the CNS. (A CNS neuron on which a primary sensory neuron synapses is called a second order neuron, which in turn synapses on a third order neuron, etc.) With few exceptions, the receptive endings, cell body and central terminals of primary sensory neurons are all on the same side. Motor neurons that innervate skeletal muscle (also called lower motor neurons) have their cell bodies within the CNS but, like primary sensory neurons, almost always are connected to ipsilateral structures.

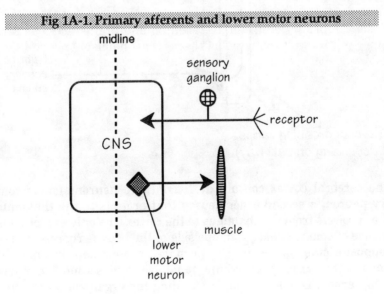

Fig 1A-1. Primary afferents and lower motor neurons

4. Sensory pathways to the cerebral cortex involve a chain of at least three neurons, the second having an axon that typically crosses the midline.

Most kinds of sensory information divide into two streams after entering the CNS (each stream being actually a series of parallel creeks in most instances). One stream is directed to the cerebral cortex, the other to the cerebellum. The information that reaches the cerebral cortex is used in our conscious awareness of the world, as well as in figuring out appropriate behavioral responses to what's going on out there. The information that reaches the cerebellum, in contrast, is used solely in motor control; someone with cerebellar dysfunction moves abnormally but has normal awareness of the abnormality.

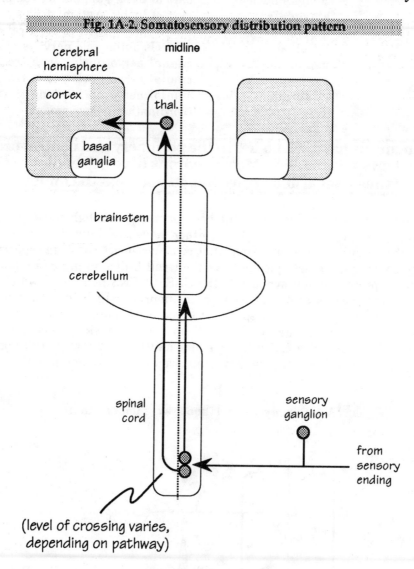

Fig. 1A-2. Somatosensory distribution pattern

Pathways to the cerebral cortex contain **at least** three neurons (some contain more): a primary sensory neuron, a second order neuron that projects to the thalamus, and a third order neuron that projects from the thalamus to the cortex (the only exception is the olfactory system). In the case of somatic sensation, one side of the body is represented in the cerebral cortex of the opposite side. Since neither primary sensory neurons nor thalamocortical neurons have axons that cross the midline, it follows that second order neurons are the ones with crossing axons. One key to understanding the organization of sensory pathways is therefore knowing the location of the second order neurons (see text Fig. 1-4, p.4). Other sensory pathways have bilateral projections at the level of second order neurons; an example is the auditory system, where sound localization requires comparison of information from the two ears.

Pathways from the periphery to the cerebellum are simpler because the thalamus is not involved. At their simplest, they contain only a primary sensory neuron and a second order neuron that projects to the cerebellum. Curiously, one side of the cerebellum is related to the same side of the body. Part of the basis for this situation is that sensory pathways to the cerebellum typically do not cross the midline.

5. Connections between the basal ganglia and the cerebral cortex are uncrossed, whereas connections between the cerebellum and the cerebral cortex are crossed.

Signals for the initiation of voluntary movements issue from the cerebral cortex. The thalamus is not a relay in pathways leaving the cerebral cortex, and there is a large corticospinal tract that projects directly from cortex to spinal cord (and an analogous corticobulbar tract that projects to cranial nerve motor nuclei). Most corticospinal fibers, consistent with the pattern in the somatosensory system, cross the midline.

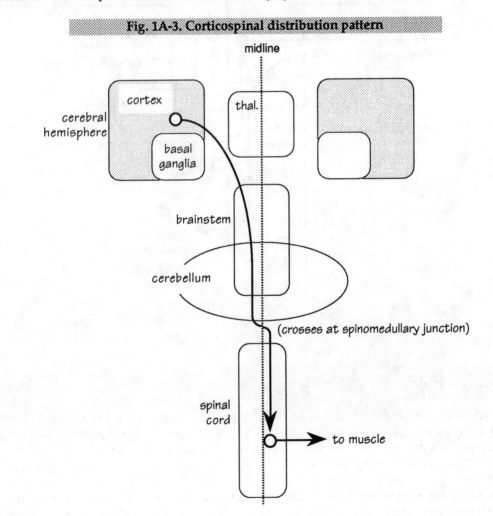

Fig. 1A-3. Corticospinal distribution pattern

6

Just as some sensory systems project bilaterally to the thalamus and cortex, some motor neurons receive bilateral innervation from the cerebral cortex. This is particularly true for motor neurons to muscles near the midline that normally work together, such as the muscles of the larynx and pharynx. Motor neurons to limb muscles, on the other hand, receive an almost entirely crossed corticospinal innervation.

The basal ganglia and the cerebellum are also involved in control of movement. However, both work not by influencing motor neurons directly, but rather by affecting the output of motor areas of the cortex. Connections between the basal ganglia and the cerebral cortex for the most part do not cross the midline, so one-sided damage to the basal ganglia causes contralateral deficits. In contrast, connections between the cerebrum and the cerebellum are crossed, consistent with the observation that one-sided cerebellar damage typically causes ipsilateral deficits. Since the cerebellum and basal ganglia affect motor but not sensory areas of the cortex, damage to the cerebellum or basal ganglia does not cause changes in basic sensation.

Fig. 1A-4. Connections of the basal ganglia and cerebellum with cerebral cortex

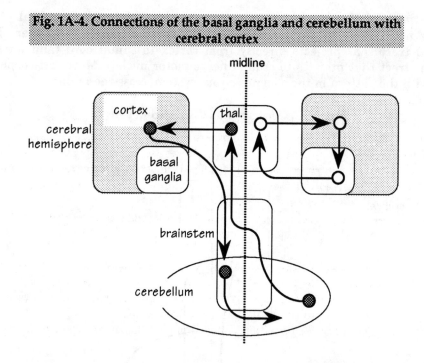

Self-Evaluation Questions

1. Which of the following is most likely to be a gray matter structure?
   a) lateral lemniscus
   b) putamen
   c) medial longitudinal fasciculus
   d) superior cerebellar peduncle

For questions 2-5, match the structures in the left column with the subdivisions of the CNS in the column on the right; a subdivision can be used once, more than once or not at all.

2. lenticular nucleus   a) cerebral hemisphere
3. pons   b) diencephalon
4. hypothalamus   c) brainstem
5. amygdala   d) cerebellum

6. The primary afferent neurons for touch in the big toe have their cell bodies in
   a) ipsilateral spinal gray matter.
   b) contralateral spinal gray matter.
   c) ipsilateral ganglia adjacent to the spinal cord.
   d) contralateral ganglia adjacent to the spinal cord.

7. The facial nerve controls the muscles used to wrinkle the forehead as well as those used for smiling. Damage to motor cortex on one side commonly causes weakness of contralateral smiling muscles but does not cause pronounced weakness of forehead muscles on either side. The most likely explanation of this observation is that
   a) each facial motor nucleus has motor neurons for the forehead muscles of both sides, but the smiling muscles of only one side.
   b) the cerebral cortex of each side sends mostly crossed projections to some facial motor neurons, and bilateral projections to other facial motor neurons.

8. Damage to a sensory area of the left cerebral cortex causes deficits on the right because
   a) primary afferents cross the midline on their way to second-order cells.
   b) second-order cells have axons that cross the midline on the way to the thalamus.
   c) thalamic neurons project to the contralateral cerebral cortex.
   d) any of the above could be responsible, depending on the sensory system involved.

9. Damage to the right side of the cerebellum causes
   a) incoordination of the right arm due to inability to perceive its position.
   b) incoordination of the left arm due to inability to perceive its position.
   c) difficulty controlling the left arm, with full awareness of its abnormal movement.
   d) difficulty controlling the right arm, with full awareness of its abnormal movement.

10. Damage to the right basal ganglia causes a left-sided movement disorder because
    a) fibers from the basal ganglia descend to the spinal cord, crossing along the way.
    b) fibers from the basal ganglia project to the contralateral thalamus, which in turn projects to the spinal cord.
    c) fibers from the basal ganglia project to the ipsilateral thalamus, which in turn sends crossed fibers to the spinal cord.
    d) the basal ganglia project to the thalamus, which in turn projects to motor cortex; these connections are all uncrossed, but motor cortex sends crossed fibers to the spinal cord.
    e) the basal ganglia project to the ipsilateral motor cortex, which in turn sends crossed fibers to the spinal cord.

Answers and Explanations

1. **b**. Lemniscus, fasciculus and peduncle all refer to white matter structures, leaving putamen as the logical choice. The putamen is in fact a large nucleus that is part of the basal ganglia.

2. **a**.

3. **c**.

4. **b**.

5. **a**.

6. **c**. See Section 3 in this chapter.

7. **b**. Since motor neurons almost always project ipsilaterally, **a** is unlikely. In fact, as explained in Chapter 9B, the explanation proposed in **b** is correct.

8. **b**. See Fig. 1A-2.

9. **d**. Cerebellar damage does not cause sensory deficits; it causes an ipsilateral movement disorder.

10. **d**. See Figs. 1A-3 and 1A-4.

CHAPTER 1B

EMBRYOLOGY OF THE CENTRAL NERVOUS SYSTEM

<u>LEARNING OBJECTIVES</u>

1. Describe the origin of neural crest cells during the development of the nervous system, and indicate the fate of these cells.

2. Name the primary and secondary embryonic vesicle from which each of the following major brain structures is derived: medulla, pons, midbrain, cerebellum, thalamus, hypothalamus, cerebral cortex, caudate nucleus, putamen and amygdala. Indicate the secondary embryonic vesicle giving rise to each of the four ventricles of the brain.

3. Describe the relationships among the alar and basal plates, the sulcus limitans, and the sensory and motor nuclei of the central nervous system. Include in your description an indication of how the dorsal/ventral relationship of the spinal alar and basal plates is altered during development of the brainstem.

4. Describe the sequence of events which leads to the formation of a C-shaped cerebrum from a linear neural tube.

Understanding a little bit about the embryology of the brain helps to clarify the way it's put together in adults. The central nervous system starts out as a simple ectodermal tube that develops some folds and bulges. The cavity of the tube persists as the ventricular system, and the folds and bulges determine the shape and layout of many parts of the CNS.

1. Neural crest cells form most of the peripheral nervous system.

Cells of the neural crest grow at the apex of each neural fold. When the neural folds fuse to form the neural tube, the neural crest becomes a detached layer between the neural tube and the surface ectoderm (text Fig. 1-6, p.6). Neural crest cells go on to form neurons and glial cells of the peripheral nervous system. These include the primary sensory neurons of spinal and most cranial ganglia, postganglionic autonomic neurons, and the Schwann cells and satellite cells of peripheral nerves and ganglia.

2. The brain develops from forebrain, midbrain, and hindbrain vesicles of the neural tube.

As the neural tube closes, it develops a series of three bulges or primary vesicles. The walls of these three vesicles go on to form the entire brain, and their continuous cavity forms the ventricular system. Since in many ways the CNS retains much of the longitudinal organization of the neural tube, these vesicles provide some useful functional terminology for different CNS regions. The most rostral primary vesicle is the prosencephalon (Greek for "front-brain" or forebrain), followed by the mesencephalon or midbrain, followed by the rhombencephalon or hindbrain, which merges with the embryonic spinal cord. The rhombencephalon is named for the rhomboid fourth ventricle which it contains.

Both the prosencephalon and rhombencephalon divide into two secondary vesicles, so there is a total of five secondary vesicles. The prosencephalon forms the telencephalon ("end-brain") and the diencephalon ("in-between-brain"). The telencephalon gives rise to the two cerebral hemispheres and its cavity becomes the lateral ventricles. The diencephalon gives rise to the thalamus, hypothalamus, retina and several other structures; its cavity becomes the third ventricle. The mesencephalon remains undivided as the midbrain; its cavity persists as the cerebral aqueduct, which interconnects the third and fourth ventricles. The rhombencephalon forms the metencephalon and the myelencephalon, which together give rise to the cerebellum and the rest of the brainstem, and enclose the fourth ventricle. All this is shown schematically in Fig. 1B-1.

3. Alar and basal plates, separated by the sulcus limitans, develop into sensory and motor nuclei.

The sulcus limitans is a longitudinal groove that develops in the lateral wall of the embryonic spinal cord and rhombencephalon. It separates two groups of neuronal cell bodies, the alar plate (dorsal to the sulcus limitans in the spinal cord) and the basal plate (ventral to the sulcus limitans in the spinal cord). The alar and basal plates go on to become sensory and motor structures, respectively. The spinal alar plate becomes the posterior horn, where primary sensory neurons terminate. The spinal basal plate becomes the anterior horn, where the cell bodies of motor neurons live.

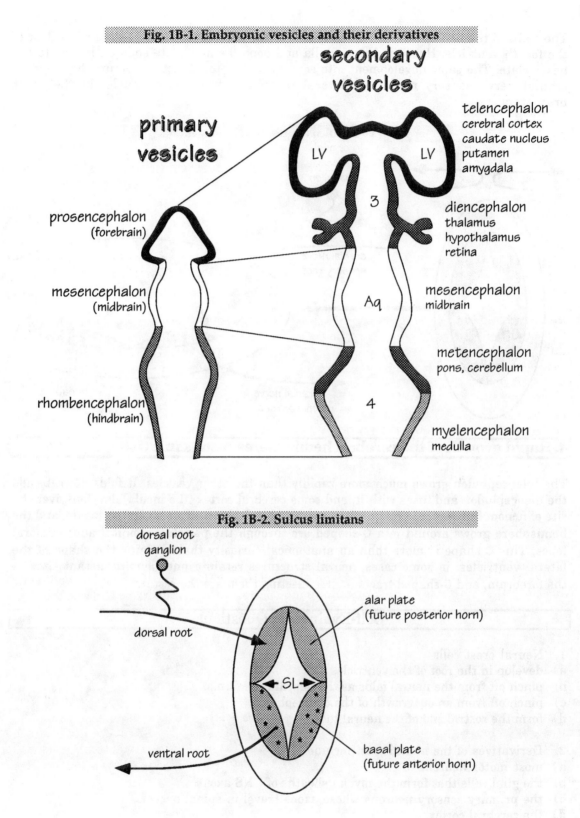

Fig. 1B-1. Embryonic vesicles and their derivatives

secondary vesicles

primary vesicles

telencephalon
cerebral cortex
caudate nucleus
putamen
amygdala

prosencephalon
(forebrain)

diencephalon
thalamus
hypothalamus
retina

mesencephalon
(midbrain)

mesencephalon
midbrain

metencephalon
pons, cerebellum

rhombencephalon
(hindbrain)

myelencephalon
medulla

LV   LV
3
Aq
4

Fig. 1B-2. Sulcus limitans

dorsal root ganglion

dorsal root

alar plate
(future posterior horn)

SL

ventral root

basal plate
(future anterior horn)

12

The walls of the neural tube are spread apart in the rhombencephalon, forming the floor of the fourth ventricle. Hence in the medulla and pons the alar plate ends up lateral to the basal plate. The same development into sensory and motor structures occurs, however, so cranial nerve sensory nuclei are lateral to cranial nerve motor nuclei in the adult brainstem.

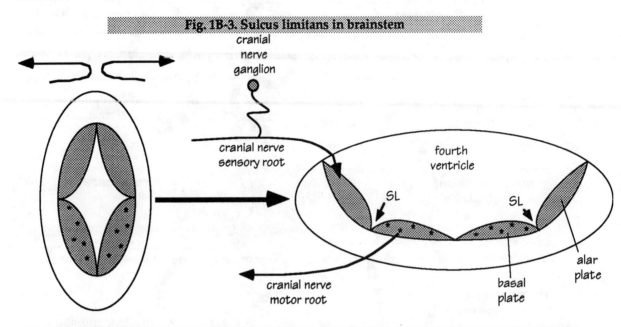

Fig. 1B-3. Sulcus limitans in brainstem

4. Rapid growth of the cerebral hemispheres results in a C shape.

The telencephalon grows much more rapidly than the other vesicles. It folds down beside the diencephalon and fuses with it, and some cerebral cortex (the insula) develops over the site of fusion. Subsequent growth of the cerebral hemisphere pivots about the insula, and the hemisphere grows around in a C-shaped arc through the parietal, occipital and temporal lobes. This C shape is more than an anatomical curiosity that explains the shape of the lateral ventricles: in some cases, neural structures retain connections to distant sites in the forebrain, and C-shaped tracts interconnecting them are the result.

Self-Evaluation Questions

1. Neural crest cells
a) develop in the roof of the ventricles.
b) pinch off from the neural folds as the neural tube forms.
c) pinch off from an outgrowth of the diencephalon.
d) form the rostral end of the neural tube.

2. Derivatives of the neural crest include
a) most motor neurons.
b) the glial cells that form the myelin sheaths of CNS axons.
c) the primary sensory neurons whose axons travel in spinal nerves.
d) the cerebral cortex.

For questions 3-5, match the structures in the column on the left with the vesicles of the neural tube in the column on the right; a vesicle can be used once, more than once or not at all.

3. thalamus
   a) prosencephalon

4. cerebellum
   b) mesencephalon

5. amygdala
   c) rhombencephalon

For questions 6-9, match the structures in the column on the left with the vesicles of the neural tube in the column on the right; a vesicle can be used more than once or not at all.

6. pons
   a) myelencephalon

7. caudate nucleus
   b) metencephalon

8. third ventricle
   c) mesencephalon

9. retina
   d) diencephalon

   e) telencephalon

10. On embryological grounds, one would expect the nucleus containing motor neurons for tongue muscles (the hypoglossal nucleus) to be located _____ to the nucleus where primary afferents from tongue touch receptors terminate.
   a) medial
   b) lateral
   c) dorsal
   d) ventral

Answers and Explanations

1. **b.**

2. **c.** The only peripheral nervous system structure on the list.

3. **a.**

4. **c.**

5. **a.**

6. **b.**

7. **e.**

8. **d.**

9. **d.**

10. **a.** See Fig. 1B-3. The hypoglossal nucleus is in fact located medial to the spinal trigeminal nucleus, where some tongue touch receptors terminate (Fig. 8-2).

CHAPTER 2

GROSS ANATOMY

LEARNING OBJECTIVES

1. Describe the location and orientation of the cephalic flexure. Indicate the implications of this flexure for the meaning of the terms dorsal, posterior and superior.

2. Define, and indicate on a drawing or photograph of a brain, the boundaries of the cerebral lobes.

3. Identify the following on a drawing or photograph of a cerebral hemisphere: central, lateral, parietooccipital and calcarine sulci; precentral and postcentral gyri; superior, middle and inferior frontal gyri; superior, middle and inferior temporal gyri; uncus; occipitotemporal and parahippocampal gyri; orbital gyri, gyrus rectus, cingulate gyrus. Indicate the approximate locations of primary motor, somatosensory, visual and auditory cortex.

4. Identify the following on a drawing or photograph of the medial surface of a hemisected brain: corpus callosum (and its parts), anterior commissure and fornix; septum pellucidum; thalamus and hypothalamus; optic chiasm; subdivisions of the brainstem; pineal gland; cerebellar hemispheres and vermis; lateral, third and fourth ventricles and cerebral aqueduct.

5. In representative coronal and horizontal brain sections, identify the following: lateral ventricle; insula; hippocampal formation, amygdala, lenticular nucleus (and its parts), caudate nucleus and thalamus; internal capsule.

A useful way to start studying the brain is to learn some of the vocabulary that refers to its major parts, and to understand in a vague way what they do. These major parts can then serve as reference points to build on.

1. The axis of the CNS bends about 100° at the midbrain-diencephalon junction.

The cephalic flexure of the embryonic neural tube persists in the adult brain as a bend of about 100° between the midbrain and the diencephalon. Terms like dorsal and ventral, however, are used as though the flexure did not exist and the CNS was still a straight tube. The result is that in the spinal cord and brainstem dorsal has the same meaning as posterior, whereas in the forebrain dorsal has the same meaning as *superior*.

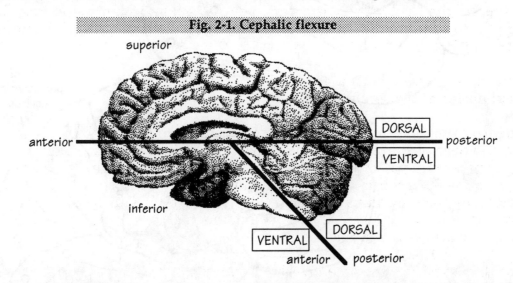

Fig. 2-1. Cephalic flexure

2. The cerebral cortex is divided into frontal, parietal, occipital and temporal lobes.

The surface of each cerebral hemisphere is wrinkled into a series of gyri separated by sulci. Three prominent sulci, together with one additional but obscure landmark, are used to divide the hemisphere into four lobes. The central sulcus forms the border between the frontal and parietal lobes. The lateral sulcus forms the border between the temporal lobe and the frontal and parietal lobes. The parietooccipital sulcus and the preoccipital notch separate the occipital lobe from the temporal and parietal lobes.

The insula, an area of cortex buried in the lateral fissure (text Fig. 2-7, p. 18), is not considered part of any of these lobes. In addition, the cingulate and parahippocampal gyri (Fig. 2-3) are often considered separately as the limbic lobe.

16

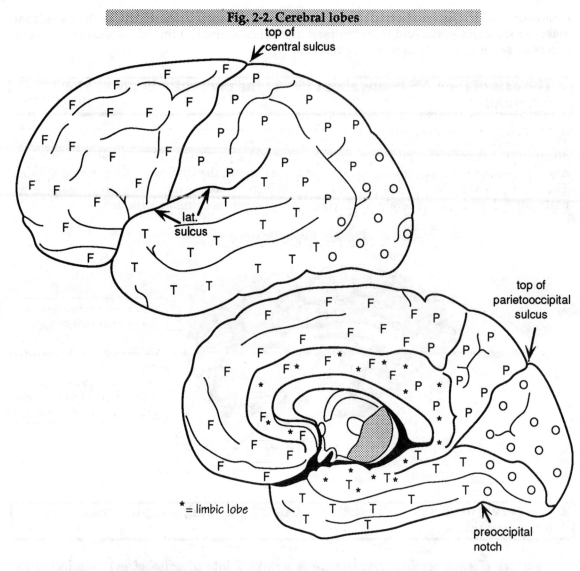

Fig. 2-2. Cerebral lobes

top of central sulcus

lat. sulcus

top of parietooccipital sulcus

preoccipital notch

*= limbic lobe

---

3. A number of fairly constant gyri and sulci are present on the cortical surface; some correspond to specific functional areas.

Frontal lobe. The lateral surface of the frontal lobe is made up of the precentral gyrus and the superior, middle and inferior frontal gyri. The precentral gyrus is located immediately in front of the central sulcus and most of it is primary motor cortex (i.e., much of the corticospinal tract originates here). The other three are broad, parallel gyri that extend anteriorly from the precentral gyrus. The precentral and superior frontal gyri extend over onto the medial surface of the frontal lobe, which is completed by a portion of the cingulate gyrus. The inferior (or orbital) surface of the frontal lobe is made up of a series of unnamed orbital gyri together with gyrus rectus, which is located adjacent to the midline.

Parietal lobe. The major named gyrus of the parietal lobe is the postcentral gyrus. The postcentral gyrus corresponds to primary somatosensory cortex (i.e., ascending somatosensory pathways terminate most heavily here) and, like the precentral gyrus, extends over onto the medial surface of the parietal lobe. Another portion of the cingulate gyrus forms an additional part of the medial surface of the parietal lobe.

Occipital lobe. The occipital lobe has no gyri with commonly used names. However, its medial surface is bisected by the calcarine sulcus, which is flanked by primary visual cortex.

Temporal lobe. The temporal lobe is covered by five long parallel gyri. The superior, middle and inferior temporal gyri are exposed on the lateral surface. The inferior temporal gyrus extends around onto the inferior surface and is followed by the occipitotemporal gyrus and the parahippocampal gyrus. At its anterior end the parahippocampal gyrus folds back on itself to form a bump called the uncus. The para-hippocampal gyrus received its name because it is continuous with a cortical region called the hippocampal formation, which is rolled into the temporal lobe and visible only in sections (Fig. 2-5). Primary auditory cortex occupies a small portion of the superior temporal gyrus, mostly in the wall of the lateral sulcus.

Fig. 2-3. Prominent gyri and sulci

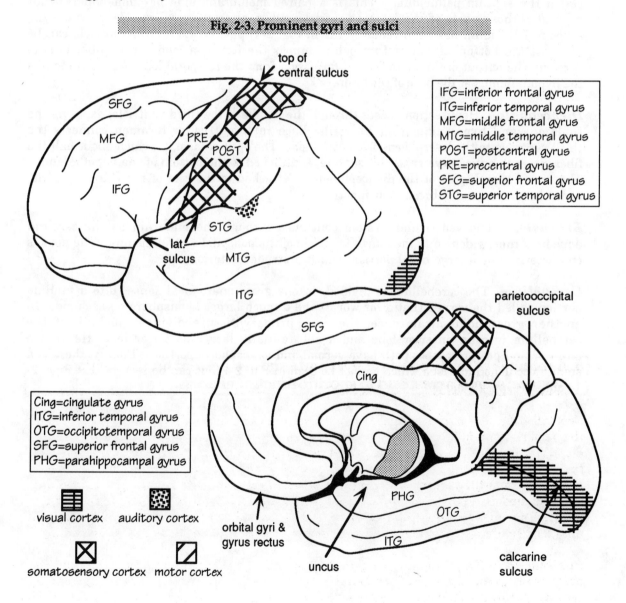

IFG=inferior frontal gyrus
ITG=inferior temporal gyrus
MFG=middle frontal gyrus
MTG=middle temporal gyrus
POST=postcentral gyrus
PRE=precentral gyrus
SFG=superior frontal gyrus
STG=superior temporal gyrus

Cing=cingulate gyrus
ITG=inferior temporal gyrus
OTG=occipitotemporal gyrus
SFG=superior frontal gyrus
PHG=parahippocampal gyrus

visual cortex   auditory cortex

somatosensory cortex   motor cortex

18

4. Hemisecting a brain reveals the ventricular system, much of the diencephalon, and the divisions of the brainstem.

The cerebral hemispheres are so big that they hide much of the rest of the brain from view. Hemisection reveals not only additional parts of the hemispheres, but also much of the diencephalon, brainstem and cerebellum.

Cerebral hemispheres. The hemispheres are interconnected by two fiber bundles. The corpus callosum extends from an enlarged genu in the frontal lobe through a body to an enlarged splenium in the parietal lobe. It interconnects the frontal, parietal and occipital lobes. The smaller anterior commissure performs a similar function for the temporal lobes. Beneath the corpus callosum in an accurately hemisected brain is a membrane called the septum pellucidum . This is a paired membrane (one per hemisphere) that separates those parts of the lateral ventricles adjacent to the midline. Hence when the septum pellucidum has been removed (as in Fig. 2-4) part of the lateral ventricle can be seen. At the bottom of the septum pellucidum is the fornix, a long curved fiber bundle carrying the output of the hippocampal formation from the temporal lobe to structures like the hypothalamus at the base of the brain.

Diencephalon. Hemisection passes through the middle of the third ventricle, exposing the thalamus and hypothalamus in its walls. Each interventricular foramen connects the third ventricle to the lateral ventricle of that side. The optic chiasm, in which about half the fibers in each optic nerve cross the midline, is attached to the bottom of the hypothalamus. The pineal gland (part of the diencephalon) is attached to the roof of the third ventricle, near the diencephalon-brainstem junction.

Brainstem. The ventricular system continues through the midbrain as the cerebral aqueduct, then widens into the fourth ventricle of the pons and rostral medulla. The pons is characterized by a large basal portion, which protrudes anteriorly.

Cerebellum. The cerebellum is divided, in one gross anatomical sense, into a midline portion called the vermis (Latin for worm) and a much larger hemisphere on each side. In another gross anatomical sense, the deep primary fissure divides the bulk of the cerebellum into an anterior lobe and a substantially larger posterior lobe. Hence the anterior and posterior lobes both have vermal and hemispheral portions. Finally, there is a small flocculonodular lobe which cannot be seen in Fig. 2-4 (but can be seen in text Figs. 2-14 and 2-16, pp. 23 and 26).

19

Fig. 2-4. Hemisected brain

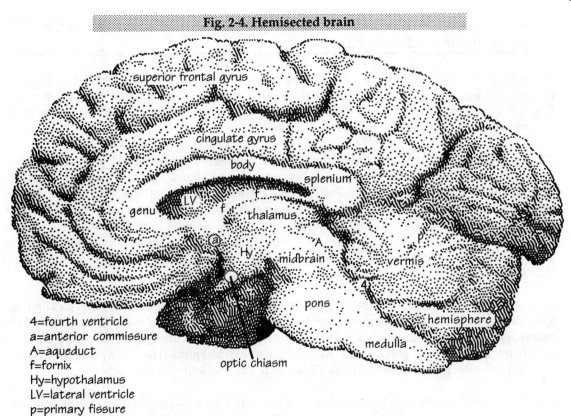

superior frontal gyrus

cingulate gyrus

body

splenium

genu LV f F

thalamus

a

Hy midbrain

A

p

vermis

pons

hemisphere

medulla

optic chiasm

4=fourth ventricle
a=anterior commissure
A=aqueduct
f=fornix
Hy=hypothalamus
LV=lateral ventricle
p=primary fissure

5. Sectioning a brain reveals the basal ganglia, hippocampal formation, amygdala and internal capsule.

A number of forebrain structures are completely enveloped by the cerebral hemispheres and cannot be seen without sectioning the brain. Coronal sections such as that shown in Fig. 2-5 reveal the general arrangement of these structures; horizontal sections such as that shown in Fig. 2-6 help to reveal their extent.

Two major components of the basal ganglia, the putamen and the globus pallidus (referred to together as the lenticular nucleus) lie beneath the insula. Another major forebrain component of the basal ganglia, the caudate nucleus, travels in the wall of the lateral ventricle. Like the lateral ventricle, the caudate nucleus is C-shaped. It extends from an enlarged head in the frontal lobe, through a body (shown in Fig. 2-5) in the frontal and parietal lobes, to a thin tail in the temporal lobe. (The tail of the caudate nucleus is actually present in the slice from which Fig. 2-5 was made, but is so small that it cannot be seen at this resolution.)

Between the lenticular nucleus and the thalamus is a thick bundle of fibers called the internal capsule; it continues anteriorly between the lenticular nucleus and the head of the caudate nucleus. The internal capsule is the principal route through which fibers travel to and from the cerebral cortex. For example, the corticospinal tract travels through the internal capsule, as do somatosensory fibers from the thalamus to the cortex.

The slice shown in Fig. 2-5 is similar to those in text Fig. 13-2 (p. 321). This particular one was cut a little asymmetrically, so that the right side of the figure is slightly anterior to the left side. On the right side underlying the uncus is a large nucleus called the amygdala, an important component of the limbic system. Just beneath it is the most anterior part of the hippocampal formation, a cortical structure that has been folded into the temporal lobe. (The left side of Fig. 2-6 is slightly posterior to the amygdala, which has been entirely replaced by the hippocampal formation.) The hippocampal formation is another major component of the limbic system.

Fig. 2-5. Coronal section of forebrain

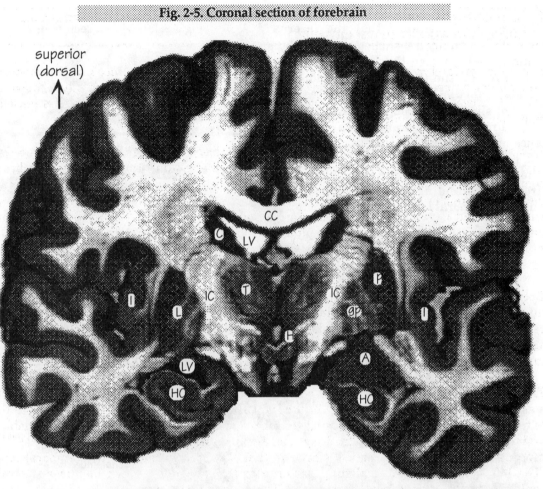

superior
(dorsal)

gp=globus pallidus
p=putamen
A=amygdala
C=caudate nucleus
CC=corpus callosum
H=hypothalamus

HC=hippocampal formation
I=insula
IC=internal capsule
L=lenticular nucleus (putamen+globus pallidus)
LV=lateral ventricle
T=thalamus

VIEW ⟶

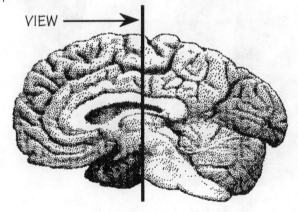

Horizontal slices show that the internal capsule is actually a **V**-shaped sheet of fibers sandwiched between the lenticular nucleus laterally and the thalamus and head of the caudate medially. Horizontal slices, like coronal slices, cut through various **C**-shaped structures of the forebrain in two places. The slice in Fig. 2-7 is similar to that in text Fig. 13-1 (p. 320); both the lateral ventricle and the caudate nucleus are cut once in the frontal lobe and again as they curve down into the temporal lobe.

Fig.2-6. Horizontal section of forebrain

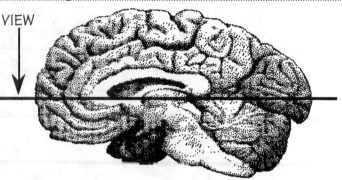

VIEW

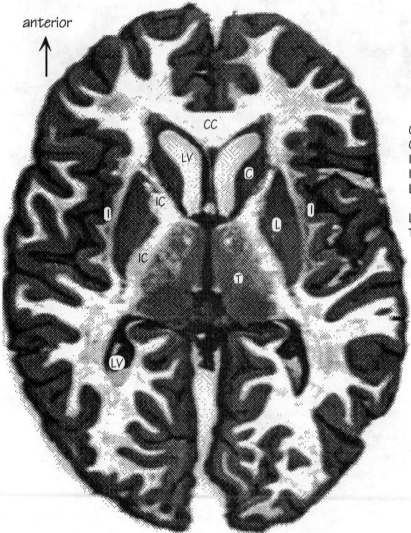

anterior

C=caudate nucleus
CC=corpus callosum
I=insula
IC=internal capsule
L=lenticular nucleus
  (putamen+globus pallidus)
LV=lateral ventricle
T=thalamus

Self-Evaluation Questions

Answer questions 1–5 using the letters on the following diagram. A letter may be used once, more than once or not at all.

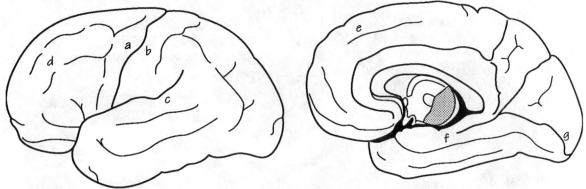

1. Somatosensory cortex
2. Superior frontal gyrus
3. Part of the parietal lobe
4. Visual cortex
5. Parahippocampal gyrus

Answer questions 6–10 using the letters on the following diagram. A letter may be used once, more than once or not at all.

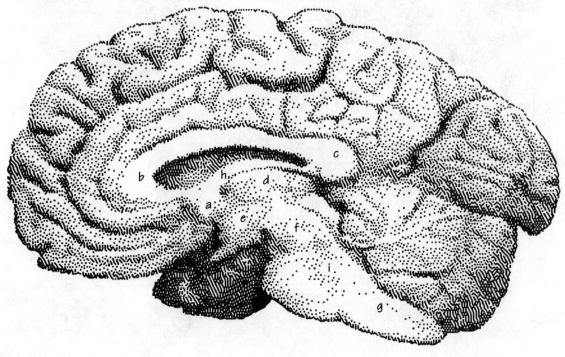

6. Pons
7. Splenium of the corpus callosum
8. Output from the hippocampal formation
9. Major relay in pathways to the cerebral cortex
10. Control center for the autonomic nervous system

24

Answer questions 11-15 using the letters on the following diagram. A letter may be used once, more than once or not at all.

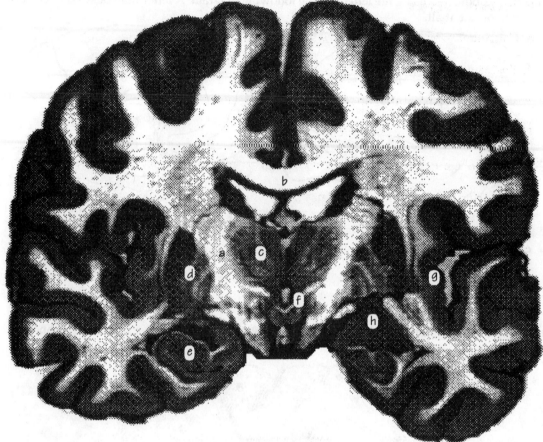

11. Insula
12. Part of the basal ganglia
13. Thalamus
14. Lenticular nucleus
15. Hippocampal formation

Answers and Explanations

1. **b**. Postcentral gyrus.

2. **e**. Continues over onto the medial surface of the hemisphere.

3. **b**. Postcentral gyrus, behind the central sulcus.

4. **g**. Visual cortex is located above and below the calcarine sulcus.

5. **f**. Most medial gyrus of the temporal lobe.

6. **i**. Between the midbrain (**f**) and medulla (**g**). Large basal portion protrudes anteriorly.

7. **c**. Posterior enlargement, containing parietal and occipital fibers.

8. **h**. The fornix.

9. **d**. The thalamus.

10. **e**. The hypothalamus.

11. **g**. Cortex buried in the lateral sulcus.

12. **d**. Lenticular nucleus (putamen + globus pallidus).

13. **c**.

14. **d**.

15. **e**. Cortical layer folded into the temporal lobe.

CHAPTER 3

MENINGES

<u>LEARNING OBJECTIVES</u>

1. List the three meningeal coverings of the cerebrum, cerebellum and brainstem and indicate in a general sense their histological structures. Define the real and potential spaces within and around these meningeal coverings.

2. Indicate the location and general configuration of the major dural septa, and the locations of the major venous sinuses.

3. Describe the role of the arachnoid as a barrier structure and as a partition between cerebrospinal fluid and venous blood.

4. Describe the way in which the meninges function together to maintain the shape and position of the central nervous system.

5. Differentiate between the cranial and spinal meninges.

The meninges form a major part of the mechanical suspension system of the central nervous system. In addition, they participate in the system of barriers that effectively isolates the extracellular spaces in the nervous system from the extracellular spaces in the rest of the body.

1. The central nervous system is surrounded by the dura mater, the arachnoid and the pia mater.

The dura mater, or dura, is a thick connective tissue membrane that also serves as the periosteum of the inside of the skull. The arachnoid and the pia mater (or pia) are much thinner collagenous membranes. The arachnoid is attached to the inside of the dura and the pia is attached to the outer surface of the CNS. Hence the only space normally present between or around the cranial meninges is subarachnoid space (not counting the venous sinuses found *within* the dura). The arrangement of spinal meninges is slightly different; see section 5 of this chapter.

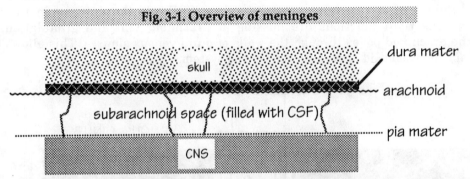

Fig. 3-1. Overview of meninges

Subarachnoid space is filled with cerebrospinal fluid (CSF), contains the arteries and veins that supply and drain the CNS, and is traversed by strands of connective tissue (arachnoid trabeculae) that interconnect the arachnoid and pia. Large pockets of subarachnoid space, corresponding to major irregularities in the surface of the CNS (see text, Fig. 3-11, p. 41), are called subarachnoid cisterns. Prominent cisterns include cisterna magna (between the medulla and the inferior surface of the cerebellum) and the superior cistern (above the midbrain).

While spaces are not normally present between the dura and either the skull or the arachnoid, these potential epidural and subdural spaces can be opened up in certain pathological conditions (text, Fig. 3-14, p. 45). Most often this is caused by tearing of a meningeal artery (→epidural bleeding) or of a cerebral vein as it enters a dural venous sinus (→subdural bleeding). Rupture of ordinary cerebral arteries and veins causes subarachnoid bleeding, since these vessels reside in subarachnoid space.

2. Infoldings of the dura mater partially divide the cranial cavity into compartments.

Inward extensions of the dura form dural reflections or dural septa. The two most prominent of these are the falx cerebri, separating the two cerebral hemispheres, and the tentorium cerebelli, separating the cerebellum and brainstem (below it) from the forebrain (above it). These are obviously not complete separations, since the two cerebral hemispheres are interconnected beneath the falx by the corpus callosum, and the brainstem continues upward through the tentorial notch into the diencephalon. The free edges of these dural reflections are the sites at which expanding masses can cause herniation of part of the brain from one compartment into another (text, Figs. 3-15 and 3-16, pp. 46 and 47).

Along some attached edges of dural reflections (and along some free edges) there is an endothelium-lined venous channel called a dural venous sinus. Prominent sinuses are the superior sagittal sinus (along the attachment of the falx cerebri to the skull), transverse sinuses (attachment of the tentorium cerebelli to the skull) and straight sinus (attachment of the falx and tentorium to each other). All four meet at the confluence of the sinuses (also called the torcular, or torcular Herophili (Greek for "the winepress of Herophilus")). Venous drainage from the brain eventually reaches these sinuses (text Fig. 5-16, p. 90).

3. The arachnoid forms a barrier between cerebrospinal fluid and the general extracellular fluids of the body.

The arachnoid includes a layer of cells that are connected to each other by bands of tight junctions, represented by dark bars in the schematic diagram below. This forms a barrier to the diffusion of extracellular substances from CSF into the dura, or in the reverse direction. The tight junctions are missing at arachnoid villi and granulations, sites where the arachnoid pokes through the walls of dural venous sinuses. This allows CSF to move from subarachnoid space into the venous system.

Fig. 3-2. Arachnoid barrier and villus

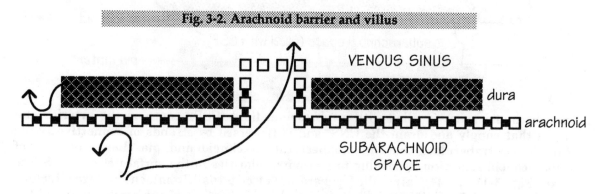

VENOUS SINUS

dura

arachnoid

SUBARACHNOID SPACE

The arachnoid barrier is part of a system, summarized in Chapter 5, that effectively separates the extracellular fluids of the nervous system from those of the rest of the body.

4. The central nervous system is stabilized in space by a combination of flotation and mechanical suspension.

The arachnoid is attached to the skull by virtue of its attachment to the dura. The pia is attached to the CNS. Hence, the arachnoid trabeculae that interconnect the pia and arachnoid form a relatively weak mechanical suspension system for the CNS. The central nervous system is completely immersed in the CSF that fills subarachnoid space. The partial flotation effect of this CSF reduces the effective weight of the CNS to the point that the meningeal suspension system can support the brain and spinal cord (see Fig. 3-3 in the next section).

5. The spinal dura mater has no periosteal component.

Spinal meninges are similar in principle to cranial meninges: thick dura lined by arachnoid, subarachnoid space filled with CSF, and suspensory interconnections between arachnoid and pia. However, at the level of the foramen magnum the periosteal component of the cranial dura continues around onto the outer surface of the skull. The result is a real spinal epidural space between the spinal dura and the vertebral periosteum (as opposed to the potential cranial epidural space, which when present is located between the periosteum and the skull).

Arachnoid trabeculae are thickened around the spinal cord to form dentate ligaments. There is a large subarachnoid cistern, the lumbar cistern, extending from vertebral levels L1/L2 to S2.

Fig. 3-3. Cranial and spinal meninges

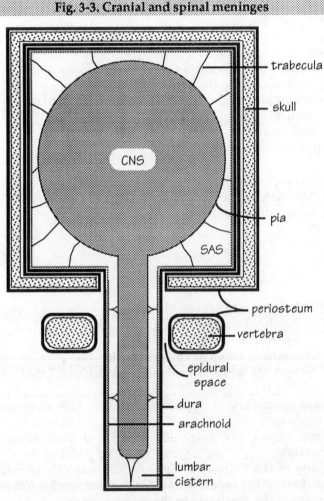

SAS=subarachnoid space

Self-Evaluation Questions

1. The thickest, mechanically strongest part of the meninges is the
   a) dura mater.
   b) arachnoid.
   c) pia mater.

2. Real spaces within the cranium include
   a) subdural space.
   b) subarachnoid space.
   c) epidural space.
   d) (a) and (b).
   e) none of the above.

3. A torn meningeal artery is most likely to cause bleeding into
   a) epidural space.
   b) subdural space.
   c) subarachnoid space.
   d) a dural venous sinus.

4. A mass in the parietal lobe might cause the ipsilateral cingulate gyrus to herniate
   a) under the falx cerebri.
   b) through the tentorial notch.
   c) past the tentorium cerebelli.
   d) none of the above.

5. A small protein molecule located in the periosteum of the skull and diffusing toward the brain would meet a diffusion barrier
   a) in the dura mater.
   b) in a layer of arachnoid cells.
   c) in the pia mater.
   d) nowhere.

6. Cerebrospinal fluid moves into venous blood by
   a) diffusing through the dural walls of venous sinuses.
   b) being actively transported across the arachnoid.
   c) passing through functional holes in the arachnoid villi.
   d) passing directly across the walls of veins in subarachnoid space.

7. All of the following are important in the maintenance of the shape and position of the CNS *except* the
   a) dentate ligaments.
   b) arachnoid trabeculae.
   c) mechanical rigidity of the CNS.
   d) partial flotation effect of the cerebrospinal fluid in subarachnoid space.
   e) physical attachment of the arachnoid to the dura.

8. One characteristic of the meninges of the spinal cord is
   a) real epidural space, between the dura and the vertebral periosteum.
   b) potential epidural space, between dura and vertebral periosteum.
   c) no subarachnoid space.
   d) a real subdural space.
   e) specialized ingrowths of the dura called dentate ligaments.

1. **a**. The name "dura" is derived from the Latin word for hard or tough (as in durable), describing this thick, collagenous membrane. The arachnoid and pia are much more delicate.

2. **b**. The cranial dura is attached to the skull externally and the arachnoid internally, so there is no real epidural or subdural space. The pia mater, on the other hand, is attached to the surface of the CNS, leaving a subarachnoid space between itself and the arachnoid.

3. **a**. Meningeal arteries reside in the periosteal part of the cranial dura, and tears in these arteries can cause separation of the dura from the cranium.

4. **a**. The cingulate gyrus, just above the corpus callosum, is adjacent to the falx cerebri (see text Fig. 3-3, p.36).

5. **b**. Cells in a particular layer of the arachnoid are connected to each other by bands of tight junctions, forming a diffusion barrier.

6. **c**. Arachnoid villi act like holes in the arachnoid barrier layer, allowing passive movement of CSF into dural venous sinuses (see text Fig. 3-12, p.42).

7. **c**. The meningeal suspension system is made necessary by the *lack* of rigidity of the CNS.

8. **a**. The spinal dura has no periosteal component, so there is a space between the spinal dura and the periosteum of the vertebrae.

CHAPTER 4

VENTRICLES AND CEREBROSPINAL FLUID

LEARNING OBJECTIVES

1. Describe the physical arrangement of the lateral, third, and fourth ventricles within the central nervous system.

2. Diagram the cellular composition of choroid plexus and indicate where choroid plexus is located within the ventricular system.

3. Describe the mechanism of production of cerebrospinal fluid and indicate in a general sense its composition.

4. Diagram the path of circulation of cerebrospinal fluid, from its site of production to its site of absorption. Describe the mechanism by which cerebrospinal fluid is returned to the venous system.

5. Define communicating and noncommunicating hydrocephalus. Give two examples of conditions causing each.

The ventricular system, the remnant of the hole in the middle of the embryonic neural tube, is an interconnected series of cavities that extends through most of the CNS. Cerebrospinal fluid is secreted within the ventricles, fills them, and flows out through three apertures to fill subarachnoid space.

1. The ventricles extend through most of the cerebral hemispheres, diencephalon and brainstem.

Each lateral ventricle is basically a **C**-shaped structure. This **C** shape curves from an inferior horn in the temporal lobe through a body in the parietal lobe and a bit of the frontal lobe, ending at the interventricular foramen where each lateral ventricle joins the third ventricle. Along this **C**-shaped course two extensions emerge from the lateral ventricle—a posterior horn that extends backward into the occipital lobe and an anterior horn that extends forward into the frontal lobe (text, Fig 4-2 A&B, pp. 50&51). The expanded area where the body and the inferior and posterior horns meet is called the atrium. Since the lateral ventricle represents the cavity of the embryonic telencephalon, telencephalic structures like the caudate nucleus and the hippocampal formation border much of it; the thalamus, a diencephalic derivative, also forms part of its floor (see text, Figs. 2-18–2-24, pp. 28–31).

The third ventricle is a midline slit in the diencephalon, with walls formed by the hypothalamus and much of the thalamus. The fourth ventricle begins rostrally at the cerebral aqueduct of the midbrain, through which it communicates with the third ventricle, and ends caudally at a mid-medullary level, where it narrows down into the vestigial central canal of the caudal medulla and the spinal cord. It reaches its widest extent at the pontomedullary junction, where it is prolonged into a lateral recess on each side. The tent-like roof of the fourth ventricle pokes up into the cerebellum.

The ventricular system communicates with subarachnoid space through three apertures of the fourth ventricle, a lateral aperture at the end of each lateral recess and a median aperture at the point where the fourth ventricle narrows down into the central canal.

2. Choroid plexus, found in all four ventricles, is a specialized pia-ependyma membrane invaginated by blood vessels.

Choroid plexus is formed at certain areas where the inner lining (i.e., ependyma) and the outer covering (i.e., pia) of the CNS are directly applied to each other, with no intervening neural tissue. At these sites, the ependymal cells are specialized to form a secretory epithelium called choroid epithelium; adjacent cells are joined by bands of tight junctions that form a diffusion barrier. Vascular connective tissue invaginates this pia/ependyma membrane, forming multiply folded choroid plexus (Fig. 4-1).

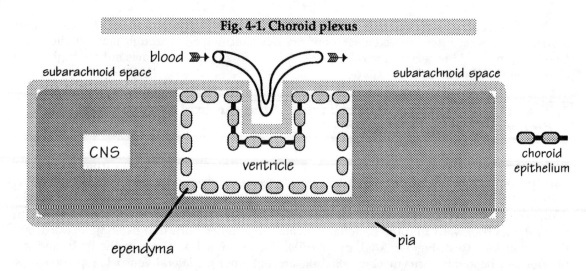

Fig. 4-1. Choroid plexus

A long strand of choroid plexus follows the **C** shape of each lateral ventricle and then grows through the interventricular foramen to become part of the roof of the third ventricle. Separate strands of choroid plexus grow in the roof of the fourth ventricle, extending laterally through the lateral apertures and caudally to the median aperture.

3. Cerebrospinal fluid is secreted by the choroid plexus.

Capillaries in the choroid plexus, unlike other capillaries inside the arachnoid barrier layer, are permeable to plasma solutes. Plasma constituents therefore leak out of these capillaries, cross the pial layer, get stopped by the choroid epithelial diffusion barrier, and form the substrate for active secretion of CSF into the ventricles by the choroid epithelium.

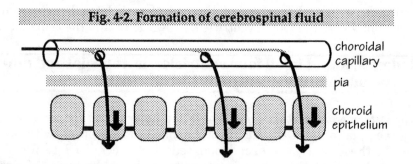

Fig. 4-2. Formation of cerebrospinal fluid

The resulting CSF is clear and colorless, low in protein, and similar (but not identical) to serum in ionic composition.

4. Cerebrospinal fluid circulates through the ventricles and subarachnoid space before moving passively into the venous system.

The cerebrospinal fluid secreted by the choroid plexuses moves through the ventricular system, pushed along by newly formed CSF. It leaves the fourth ventricle through the lateral and median apertures, moves through subarachnoid space until it reaches the arachnoid villi (which protrude primarily into the superior sagittal sinus), and finally joins the venous circulation.

Fig. 4-3. Circulation of cerebrospinal fluid

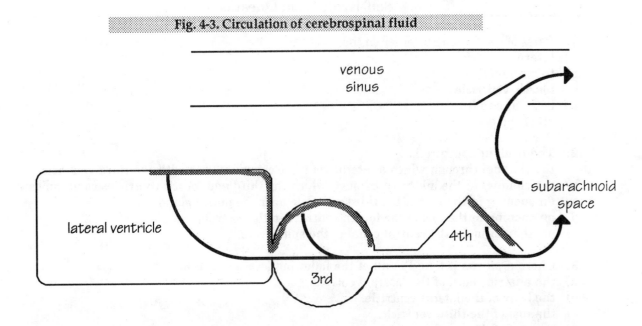

Movement across the arachnoid villi is passive, driven by the difference in hydrostatic pressure between the CSF in subarachnoid space and the venous blood in the superior sagittal sinus. The villi act like tiny flap valves, so that reverse flow is prevented if venous pressure exceeds CSF pressure.

Fig. 4-4. Arachnoid villi

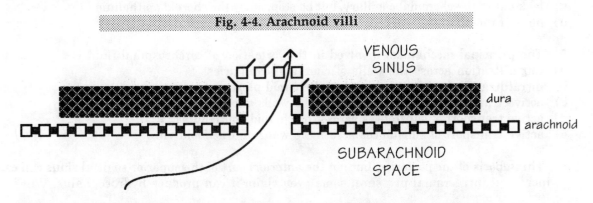

5. Obstruction of the path of CSF circulation causes hydrocephalus.

There are bottlenecks in the path of CSF circulation, both inside and outside the ventricular system. If circulation is obstructed, CSF production continues unabated and hydrocephalus results. If the obstruction cuts off the communication between some part of the ventricular system and subarachnoid space, the hydrocephalus is termed noncommunicating. If all parts of the ventricular system still communicate with at least some portion of subarachnoid space, the hydrocephalus is termed communicating. Noncommunicating hydrocephalus would be caused by processes that occluded an interventricular foramen, the aqueduct, or all three apertures of the fourth ventricle. Communicating hydrocephalus could be caused by obstruction of the tentorial notch (since CSF must pass through the notch on its way from the posterior fossa to the superior sagittal sinus) or the arachnoid villi; it could also be caused, at least theoretically, by overproduction of CSF.

1. Parts of the thalamus border on the
a) lateral ventricle.
b) third ventricle.
c) fourth ventricle.
d) both (a) and (b).
e) all of the above.

2. The median aperture is
a) the channel through which a lateral ventricle communicates with the third ventricle
b) the channel in the midbrain through which the third and fourth ventricles communicate.
c) an opening in the roof of the third ventricle near the pineal gland.
d) an opening in the roof of the fourth ventricle in the rostral pons.
e) another term for the central canal of the spinal cord.

3. Choroid plexus is found in all of the following locations *except*
a) the anterior horn of the lateral ventricle.
b) the body of the lateral ventricle.
c) the roof of the third ventricle.
d) the roof of the fourth ventricle.

4. A lipid-insoluble dye injected into an artery supplying choroid plexus would
a) not be able to leak out of the choroidal capillaries.
b) leak across the choroid plexus, but be stopped by the ependymal lining of the ventricle
c) leak out of the choroidal capillary, but be stopped by the choroid epithelium.
d) none of the above.

5. The principal mechanism involved in the formation of cerebrospinal fluid is
a) ultrafiltration across the walls of choroidal capillaries.
b) ultrafiltration across the pial layer of choroid plexus.
c) active transport of substances across the walls of choroidal capillaries.
d) active transport of substances across the choroid epithelium.
e) active transport of substances across the walls of arachnoid villi.

6. Thrombosis of the posterior (but not the anterior) part of the superior sagittal sinus can cause increased intracranial pressure; some even claim it can produce hydrocephalus. Why?

7. Noncommunicating hydrocephalus could be caused by
a) obstruction of the tentorial notch.
b) obstruction of all three apertures of the fourth ventricle.
c) obstruction of the cerebral aqueduct.
d) any of the above.
e) (b) or (c).

8. Cerebrospinal fluid leaves subarachnoid space primarily by
a) active transport across the walls of cerebral veins.
b) active transport across arachnoid villi.
c) diffusing through open channels in arachnoid villi; increased venos pressure can block this flow and force blood backward into subarachnoid space.
d) being pushed by hydrostatic pressure through arachnoid villi, in one-way bulk flow.
e) none of the above.

Answers and Explanations

1. **d.** See text Figs. 2-20 and 2-21, p. 29.

2. **d.** The median aperture and the two lateral apertures are openings in the fourth ventricle, and are the routes through which the ventricular system communicates with subarachnoid space.

3. **a.** Choroid plexus is found in all four ventricles. However, in each lateral ventricle it grows as a single **C**-shaped strand extending from the inferior horn through the body and then growing through the interventricular foramen. None grows in the anterior horn of the lateral ventricle.

4. **c.** Choroid epithelial cells are joined to one another by tight junctions, forming a diffusion barrier.

5. **d.** The choroid epithelium is a layer of ependymal cells specialized as a secretory epithelium. Substances that leak across the endothelial and pial layers of the choroid plexus are then actively transported across the choroid epithelium.

6. Arachnoid villi are the principal route through which CSF reaches the venous system, and most are located in the walls of the superior sagittal sinus. Anterior occlusions allow CSF to reach most of the villi, but posterior occlusions effectively block this normal route of CSF circulation.

7. **e.** **b** and **c** both block normal CSF circulation and cause hydrocephalus; in both cases at least part of the ventricular system is cut off from subarachnoid space. **a** also blocks CSF flow and causes hydrocephalus, but in this case the entire ventricular system is still in communication with subarachnoid space; hence **a** would cause *communicating* hydrocephalus.

8. **d.** Arachnoid villi act like flap valves inserted in the arachnoid barrier layer, allowing passive flow of CSF into the superior sagittal sinus, but not allowing flow in the opposite direction.

CHAPTER 5

BLOOD SUPPLY

LEARNING OBJECTIVES

1. Describe the general pattern of arterial supply to the cerebral hemispheres, diencephalon, brainstem and cerebellum.

2. Draw and label the circle of Willis, and discuss its functional significance.

3. Give at least two examples of mechanisms involved in the regulation of CNS blood flow.

4. List the anatomical barriers interposed between the extracellular spaces around CNS neurons and the general extracellular spaces of the body. Describe or diagram the way in which these barriers in combination isolate the extracellular spaces of the nervous system from the extracellular spaces outside the nervous system.

5. Describe the general arrangement of the superficial and deep veins of the brain.

The central nervous system is tremendously active metabolically—relative to its weight it uses much more than its share of the available oxygen and glucose. Corresponding to this metabolic activity, it has an abundant and closely regulated arterial supply and a large venous drainage system. Also, the CNS depends for its proper functioning on carefully controlled extracellular ion concentrations. Part of the basis for this control is a system of diffusion barriers of which cerebral blood vessels are a major part.

1. The internal carotid system and the vertebral-basilar system provide the blood supply to the brain.

Two interconnected arterial systems provide the blood supply to the brain. The internal carotid system of each side supplies the ipsilateral cerebral hemisphere, except for the medial surface of the occipital lobe and the inferior surface of the temporal lobe. The vertebral/basilar system supplies those parts of the occipital and temporal lobes, as well as the brainstem and cerebellum. The supply of the diencephalon is shared by the two systems, with the vertebral/basilar system supplying most of the thalamus and the internal carotid system supplying most of the hypothalamus.

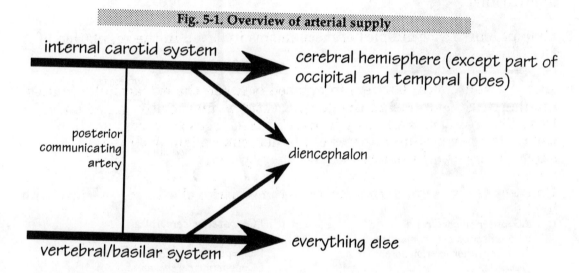

Fig. 5-1. Overview of arterial supply

The internal carotid has only two major branches, the anterior and middle cerebral arteries. The vertebral and basilar arteries have a series of branches spread out along the brainstem. The major branches in both systems have large terminal areas of distribution that are suggested to some extent by the name of the artery. For example, a posterior cerebral artery supplies posterior parts of a cerebral hemisphere. In addition, each of these major branches gives off small ganglionic or penetrating arteries along the way. These ganglionic arteries, indicated by little curved arrows in the right half of Fig. 5-2, supply the brainstem and diencephalon.

40

Fig. 5-2. Arterial supply of the brain

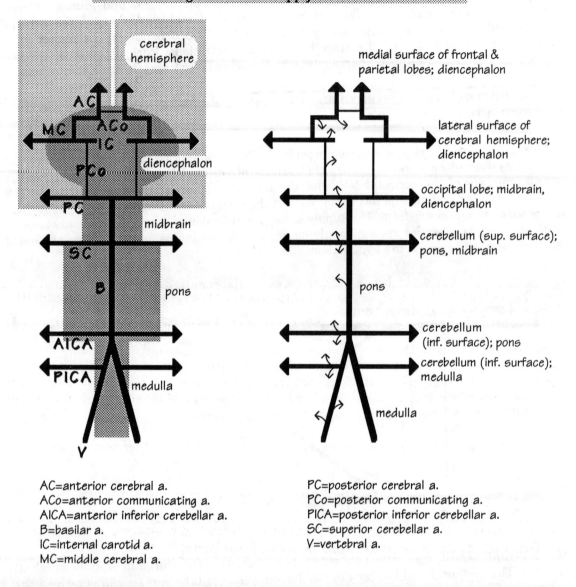

cerebral hemisphere

AC
MC
ACo
IC
PCo
diencephalon
PC
midbrain
SC
B
pons
AICA
PICA
medulla
V

medial surface of frontal & parietal lobes; diencephalon

lateral surface of cerebral hemisphere; diencephalon

occipital lobe; midbrain, diencephalon

cerebellum (sup. surface); pons, midbrain

pons

cerebellum (inf. surface); pons

cerebellum (inf. surface); medulla

medulla

AC=anterior cerebral a.
ACo=anterior communicating a.
AICA=anterior inferior cerebellar a.
B=basilar a.
IC=internal carotid a.
MC=middle cerebral a.

PC=posterior cerebral a.
PCo=posterior communicating a.
PICA=posterior inferior cerebellar a.
SC=superior cerebellar a.
V=vertebral a.

2. The circle of Willis is an anastomotic network at the base of the brain that interconnects the internal carotid and the vertebral-basilar systems.

The internal carotid and vertebral/basilar systems are interconnected by a posterior communicating artery on each side. In addition, the two anterior cerebral arteries are interconnected by the anterior communicating artery. These communicating arteries complete the arterial circle of Willis.

The communicating arteries are ordinarily fairly small and not capable of carrying much blood. However, in cases of slowly developing occlusions they can enlarge and provide a major alternative pathway for blood flow.

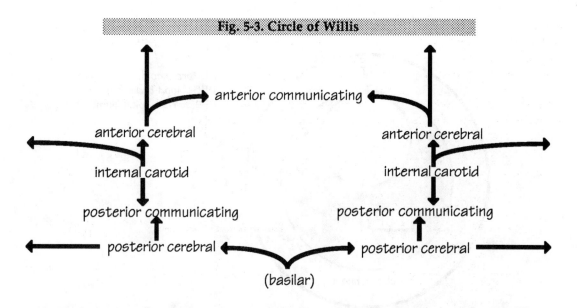

Fig. 5-3. Circle of Willis

3. CNS blood flow is automatically regulated to compensate for changes in blood flow and neural activity.

The total blood flow to the CNS, unlike that to most other organs, stays nearly constant no matter how you use your brain. Flow is maintained during changes in blood pressure by a process of autoregulation. If blood pressure drops, cerebral arterioles dilate; this compensates for the loss of pressure and lets the same amount of blood through. Conversely, if blood pressure rises, cerebral arterioles constrict.

Even though total flow to the brain remains constant, more of this flow goes to areas of the brain that are active at any given moment. This is a local response to changes in extracellular metabolites (see text, Plates 11–13). There is also autonomic innervation of cerebral vessels, but the physiological significance of this innervation is not clear.

4. A system of three barriers isolates the extracellular spaces of the CNS from the general extracellular spaces of the body.

The arachnoid barrier layer (Chapter 3) prevents things from diffusing into subarachnoid space from outside the CNS. The choroid epithelium (Chapter 4) regulates what gets into newly formed cerebrospinal fluid. The last part of the barrier system between the CNS and the rest of the body is an array of tight junctions between the endothelial cells of CNS capillaries. This blood-brain barrier prevents substances from diffusing out of CNS capillaries and allows the endothelial cells to regulate what gets into CNS extracellular space. Collectively these three barriers (Fig. 5-4) make up a system that separates the extracellular spaces of the CNS from the general extracellular spaces of the body.

Fig. 5-4. Brain barrier systems

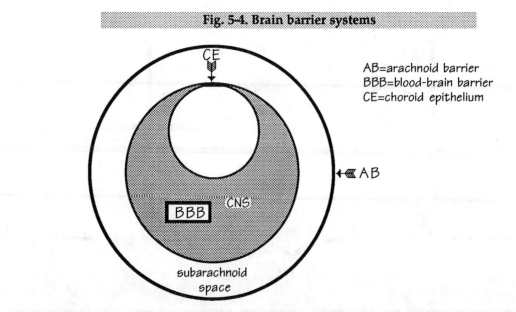

Fig. 5-4. Brain barrier systems

AB=arachnoid barrier
BBB=blood-brain barrier
CE=choroid epithelium

5. Complementary sets of superficial and deep veins drain the brain.

Two sets of veins cooperate in the drainage of the brain. Superficial veins, as their name implies, lie on the surface of each cerebral hemisphere and mostly drain upward or backward into the superior sagittal sinus. Deep veins, in contrast, converge on the internal cerebral veins above the roof of the third ventricle (text, Fig. 4-6C, p. 57).

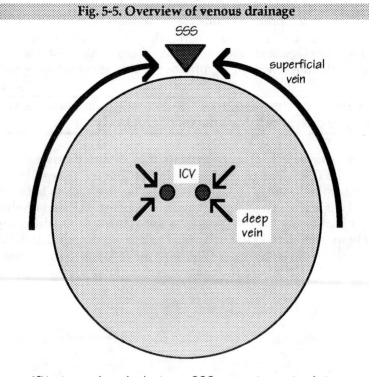

Fig. 5-5. Overview of venous drainage

ICV = internal cerebral veins   SSS = superior sagittal sinus

The two internal cerebral veins join to form the great cerebral vein (of Galen) which then joins the straight sinus. The superficial and deep drainage systems meet at the confluence of the sinuses, where the superior sagittal and straight sinuses join each other. From here, blood flows into the transverse sinuses and then reaches the sigmoid sinuses and the internal jugular veins.

Fig. 5-6. Superficial and deep veins

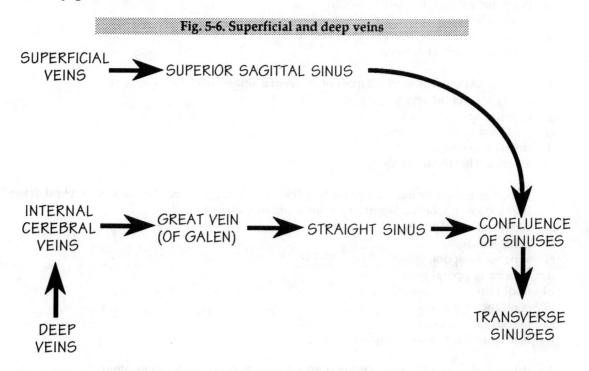

Self-Evaluation Questions

1. The caudal pons receives much of its blood supply from the
   a) vertebral artery.
   b) posterior inferior cerebellar artery.
   c) anterior inferior cerebellar artery.
   d) superior cerebellar artery.
   e) posterior cerebral artery.

2. The cingulate gyrus receives most of its arterial supply from branches of the
   a) anterior cerebral artery.
   b) middle cerebral artery.
   c) posterior cerebral artery.
   d) superior cerebellar artery.
   e) anterior choroidal artery.

3. Which of the following receive most of their blood supply from the middle cerebral artery? If any do not, which other artery is involved in each instance?
   a) superior frontal gyrus
   b) gyrus rectus
   c) superior temporal gyrus
   d) inferior temporal gyrus
   e) midbrain
   f) postcentral gyrus
   g) precentral gyrus
   h) medial surface of the occipital lobe

4. What clinical symptoms would you expect from a blood clot midway along the right posterior communicating artery? What would happen if the left posterior communicating artery became occluded sometime later?

5. The circle of Willis includes parts of all of the following *except* the
   a) internal carotid artery.
   b) posterior cerebral artery.
   c) middle cerebral artery.
   d) anterior cerebral artery.
   e) posterior communicating artery.

6. An erythrocyte travelling from a distal branch of the middle cerebral artery to the internal jugular vein would traverse all of the following *except* the
   a) superior sagittal sinus.
   b) internal cerebral vein.
   c) confluence of the sinuses.
   d) transverse sinus.

7. A lipid-insoluble dye injected into a lateral ventricle would do all of the following *except*
   a) cross the ependymal lining of the ventricle and diffuse between CNS neurons.
   b) move through the ventricular system, out into subarachnoid space, and across arachnoid villi, finally entering venous blood.
   c) diffuse across the epithelial lining of the choroid plexus and enter choroidal capillaries.
   d) be stopped by tight junctions between the endothelial cells of cerebral capillaries.

45

e) be stopped by tight junctions between arachnoid cells.

8. Sites where small protein molecules would meet a major diffusion barrier include
a) capillaries in the choroid plexus.
b) the pia mater over the surface of the brain.
c) a layer of cells in the arachnoid.
d) all of the above.
e) none of the above.

9. A 39-year-old handball hustler sat down in the corner of the court to take a break after beating 17 consecutive opponents. He started to watch a handball rolling across the court. A budding neurologist in the stands told a companion that the total blood flow to the handball hustler's brain didn't change much when he started watching the ball; instead, it increased in some areas (e.g., visual areas) and decreased in others. Was this correct?
a) yes
b) no

46

1. **c.** The vertebral and posterior inferior cerebellar arteries contribute to the supply of the medulla, the superior cerebellar and posterior cerebral arteries to the rostral pons and midbrain. See Fig. 5-2.

2. **a.** The anterior cerebral artery and its branches parallel the corpus callosum, supplying the cingulate gyrus and the medial surface of the frontal and parietal lobes.

3. a. split between anterior and middle cerebral.
   b. anterior cerebral.
   c.
   d. mostly posterior cerebral
   e. mostly posterior cerebral and superior cerebellar.
   f. (also a little from the anterior cerebral.)
   g. (also a little from the anterior cerebral.)
   h. posterior cerebral.

4. There might be no effect in either case, since under normal circumstances little blood flows through either artery. If ganglionic branches of one or both communicating arteries were involved, some deficits due to diencephalic damage might be noted.

5. **c.** See Fig. 5-3.

6. **b.** Distal branches of the middle cerebral artery are distributed to the lateral surface of the hemisphere and feed into the system of superficial veins. The internal cerebral vein is part of the system of deep veins.

7. **c.** The choroid epithelium is a diffusion barrier.

8. **c.** Choroidal capillaries, unlike usual CNS capillaries, are fenestrated; the pia mater is freely permeable at all locations.

9. **a.** Autoregulation keeps the total blood flow to the brain relatively constant. Local metabolic changes result in increased flow to active areas balanced by decreased flow to relatively inactive areas.

CHAPTER 6

SENSORY RECEPTORS AND PERIPHERAL NERVOUS SYSTEM

LEARNING OBJECTIVES

1. Define the terms "adequate stimulus" and "receptor potential".

2. Describe the physiological differences between receptors with and without long axons.

3. Differentiate between slowly adapting and rapidly adapting receptors. Indicate how receptors encode the duration and intensity of stimuli.

4. Describe the structural and functional characteristics of muscle spindles and Golgi tendon organs.

5. Tabulate the relationships between fiber size, conduction velocity, degree of myelination and sensory modality for somatic sensory fibers.

6. Tabulate the relationships between fiber size, conduction velocity and degree of myelination for somatic and autonomic efferent fibers.

7. Diagram a typical peripheral nerve, indicating the location and the general structure and function of the epineurium, perineurium and endoneurium.

48

Neural traffic to and from the CNS travels in peripheral nerves. Some constituent axons of these peripheral nerves either end as sensory receptors or carry information from sensory receptors. The others end on muscle fibers, autonomic ganglia or glands.

1. Receptors produce slow potential changes in response to particular kinds of stimuli.

Receptors are specialized cells, usually neurons, that are able to *transduce* some kind of stimulus energy into a slow electrical signal called a receptor potential (slow, that is, compared to an action potential). A given kind of receptor responds best to a particular kind of stimulus, termed the adequate stimulus for that receptor type. Photoreceptors, for example, respond best to photons.

2. Some receptors are neurons with long axons, while others have short axons (or no axons) and produce no action potentials.

Receptor potentials are not propagated actively; rather, they decay over a short distance. Therefore, receptors that signal over long distances must generate action potentials as

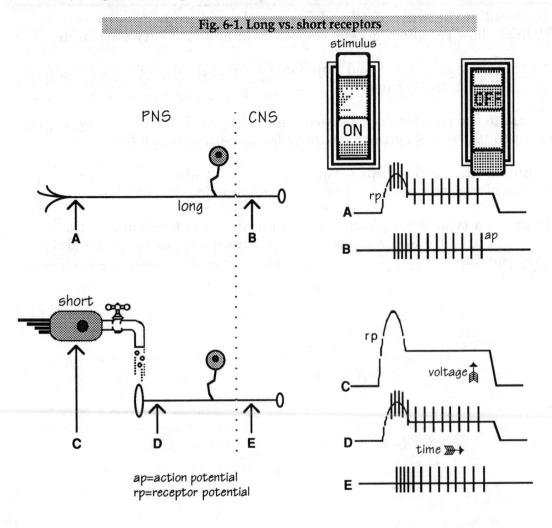

Fig. 6-1. Long vs. short receptors

ap=action potential
rp=receptor potential

well as receptor potentials. An example is a receptor that signals something touching your big toe. It produces a depolarizing receptor potential in response to touch, and the receptor potential in turn causes action potentials that are conducted all the way into the central nervous system. The receptor potential itself dies out near the receptive ending. In mammals, receptors with long axons convey information about somatic sensation (touch, pain, etc.), visceral sensation or smell, and all produce depolarizing receptor potentials.

In contrast, receptors that signal over short distances (a few mm or less) don't need to produce action potentials. Instead, they synapse on the peripheral processes of primary afferent neurons whose cell bodies lie in peripheral ganglia. The receptor potential changes the rate at which the receptor releases transmitter, and this in turn changes the rate at which the primary afferent neuron sends action potentials into the CNS. A receptor with a short axon or no axon can depolarize (and release more transmitter) or hyperpolarize (and release less transmitter) in response to a stimulus; some can do both, depending on the nature of the stimulus. Examples of short receptors are taste receptor cells, photoreceptors and hair cells of the inner ear.

3. Some receptors signal the intensity of a stimulus, while others signal its rate of change.

Some receptors produce a maintained response to a constant stimulus, and so are called slowly adapting. The response of others declines and may disappear entirely during a constant stimulus; these are called rapidly adapting. Rapidly adapting receptors can therefore act like miniature differentiators, producing a constant response to a steadily changing stimulus. The classic example of a rapidly adapting receptor is the pacinian corpuscle.

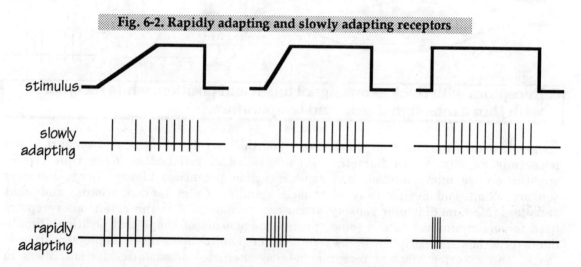

Fig. 6-2. Rapidly adapting and slowly adapting receptors

Most receptors, like the two shown in Fig.6-1, are actually somewhere between the extremes of slowly and rapidly adapting. The response may be exaggerated at the beginning (or end) of a stimulus, but maintained to some extent throughout the stimulus.

4. Muscle spindles signal the length of a muscle, while Golgi tendon organs signal its tension.

Muscle spindles are receptor organs composed of small muscle fibers (called intrafusal fibers, meaning "inside the spindle") enclosed in a spindle-shaped capsule. The spindles are embedded in skeletal muscles and oriented so that they are stretched by anything that stretches the muscle. Sensory endings applied to the intrafusal fibers produce depolarizing receptor potentials when the spindles are stretched. The ends of intrafusal fibers are contractile and receive inputs from small (gamma) motor neurons. Contraction of this part of an intrafusal fiber does not contribute significantly to the strength of a muscle. Rather, it regulates the length of the central, stretch-sensitive portion of the intrafusal fiber and thereby regulates its sensitivity to externally applied stretch (text Fig. 6-8, p.110).

Golgi tendon organs are networks of sensory endings interspersed among the collagen fibers of tendons. Tension in a tendon compresses the sensory endings and causes depolarizing receptor potentials. Passive muscle stretch does not generate much tension in a tendon, but muscle contraction against a load does.

Fig. 6-3. Muscle spindles and Golgi tendon organs

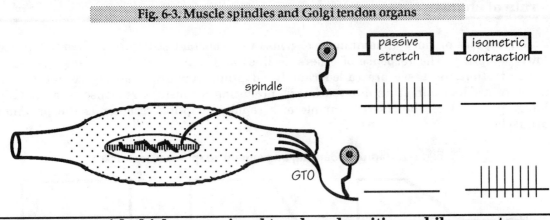

5. Receptors with thick axons signal touch and position, while receptors with thin axons signal pain and temperature.

Large-diameter axons have large cell bodies and thick myelin sheaths, and conduct action potentials rapidly. Small-diameter axons have small cell bodies, have thin myelin sheaths or are unmyelinated, and conduct action potentials slowly. Large-diameter sensory axons end peripherally in muscle spindles, Golgi tendon organs, and joint receptors. Medium-diameter sensory axons end peripherally as the cutaneous receptors used for discriminative tactile sense (precise judgements of shape and position). Small-diameter axons end peripherally as receptors for pain, temperature, simple sensation of touch, and assorted visceral receptors. Major categories of somatic afferent fibers in peripheral nerves are indicated below (see text, Table 3, p. 115, for more details).

Diameter	Myelin	Velocity	Receptors	Terms
Large	Thick	Rapid	Muscle spindles	Ia
			Golgi tendon organs	Ib
Medium	Medium	Medium	Skin, muscles, joints	II
Small	Thin	Slow	Pain, temperature, touch	delta (δ)
Smallest	None	Slow	Pain, temperature	C

6. Somatic motor neurons have relatively thick axons, while autonomic neurons have relatively thin axons.

Efferent axons of different diameters are also associated with different functions. The largest myelinated axons innervate ordinary skeletal muscle. Those that innervate intrafusal fibers are smaller, and preganglionic autonomic fibers are smaller still. Postganglionic autonomic fibers are unmyelinated.

Diameter	Myelin	Velocity	Destination/Type	Terms
Large	Thick	Rapid	Skeletal muscle	alpha (α)
Medium	Medium	Medium	Muscle spindles	gamma (γ)
Small	Thin	Slow	Preganglionic autonomic	
Smallest	None	Slow	Postganglionic autonomic	

7. Extensions of the meninges surround peripheral nerves.

The dura mater surrounding the CNS continues as the epineurium of peripheral nerves. This is a substantial covering around each nerve, conferring considerable mechanical strength. The arachnoid continues as the perineurium covering individual nerve fascicles. Perineurial cells are interconnected by tight junctions and form a diffusion barrier between the inside and the outside of a nerve fascicle. The endoneurium is the loose background connective tissue within nerve fascicles.

Fig. 6-4. Wrappings of peripheral nerves

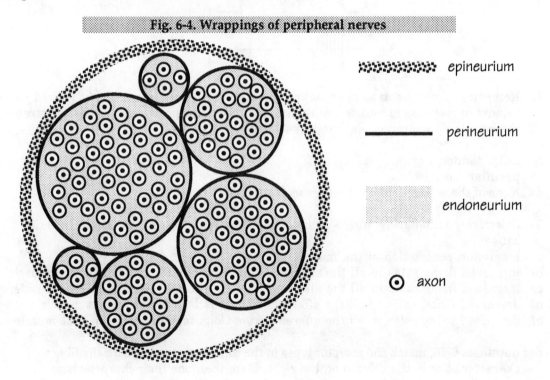

epineurium

perineurium

endoneurium

axon

52

1. The term "adequate stimulus" refers to
a) any stimulus that causes a particular receptor to increase the rate at which it produces action potentials.
b) any stimulus that causes a particular receptor to depolarize.
c) any stimulus that elicits the largest possible response from a particular receptor.
d) the kind of stimulus to which a particular receptor is most sensitive.

2. Receptors with long axons
a) produce receptor potentials that are actively propagated to the central nervous system.
b) produce receptor potentials that decay passively, but change the rate at which the receptor generates action potentials.
c) in mammals, produce depolarizing receptor potentials and increased rates of action potentials.
d) None of the above is true.
e) Both (b) and (c) are true.

3. A receptor with the following stimulus-response properties would be classified as
a) slowly adapting.
b) rapidly adapting.

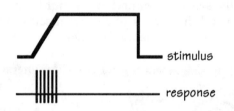

4. Recordings from the axon of an unknown muscle receptor indicated that it fired more rapidly in response to muscle contraction, but did not respond much to passive stretch of the muscle. The receptor was most likely to be a
a) muscle spindle.
b) Golgi tendon organ.
c) pacinian corpuscle.
d) None of these receptors has these response properties.

5. Selectively stimulating all the gamma motor neurons to a muscle would *initially* cause
a) maximum contraction of the muscle.
b) increased firing rates in all the afferent fibers from muscle spindles in that muscle.
c) increased firing rates in all the afferents from Golgi tendon organs in that muscle.
d) decreased firing rates in all the afferents from muscle spindles in that muscle.
e) decreased firing rates in all the afferents from Golgi tendon organs in that muscle.

For questions 6-10, match the receptor types in the column on the left with the fiber characteristics in the column on the right. More than one fiber characteristic may apply to one receptor; indicate all that apply.

6. afferents from Golgi tendon organs   a) large diameter
7. afferents from most touch receptors   b) small diameter
8. motor axons to ordinary skeletal muscle   c) heavily myelinated
9. afferents from many pain receptors   d) unmyelinated
10. postganglionic autonomic axons   e) none of the above

11. Most of the mechanical strength of peripheral nerves is a property of the
a) axons themselves.
b) epineurium.
c) perineurium.
d) endoneurium.

12. A diffusion barrier between the extracellular spaces inside and outside peripheral nerve fascicles is located
a) in the perineurium.
b) in the epineurium.
c) in the endoneurium.
d) nowhere.

Answers and Explanations

1. **d.**

2. **e.** See Section 2 in this chapter.

3. **b.** Notice that the receptor responds vigorously while the stimulus is changing, but stops responding when the stimulus is constant.

4. **b.** See Fig. 6-3.

5. **b.** Stimulating gamma motor neurons causes contraction of the ends of intrafusal fibers. This in turn stretches the central part of the intrafusal fibers, where the stretch receptor endings are applied, and makes the primary afferents fire faster. See text Fig. 6-7, p. 109.

6. **a, c.**

7. **e.** Most touch receptors are medium diameter. (See Section 5 in this chapter.)

8. **a, c.**

9. **b, d.** (Although some are thinly myelinated, many are unmyelinated.)

10. **b, d.**

11. **b.** The epineurium is continuous with the dura mater, and shares its mechanical strength.

12. **a.** The perineurium is continuous with the arachnoid, and contains a continuation of the arachnoid barrier layer.

CHAPTER 7

SPINAL CORD

LEARNING OBJECTIVES

1. Draw a schematic cross section of the spinal cord, indicating the posterior, lateral and anterior funiculi and the posterior and anterior horns. Indicate the locations of the substantia gelatinosa, the intermediolateral cell column, the dorsolateral fasciculus (Lissauer's tract) and the attachment points of the dorsal and ventral roots; briefly describe the contents and function of each.

2. Diagram a longitudinal section of the spinal cord, indicating the location of the conus medullaris, the cauda equina, the number of each type of segment, the positions of the enlargements and the relative positions of spinal nerves and vertebral segments.

3. Compare and contrast the stretch reflex and the flexor reflex in terms of function and connectivity.

4. Differentiate between the efferent connections that control skeletal muscle and those that control smooth muscle and glands.

5. Differentiate between the sympathetic and parasympathetic divisions of the autonomic nervous system.

6. Diagram the major pathway by which information from the body about touch and limb position reaches consciousness.

7. Diagram the major pathway by which information from the body about pain and temperature reaches consciousness.

8. Diagram the major pathway by which voluntary movement of the trunk and limbs is mediated.

9. In a schematic cross section of the spinal cord, identify the location and describe the contents of fasciculus gracilis, fasciculus cuneatus, the spinothalamic tract and the lateral corticospinal tract. Include in your description an indication of the origin and termination of the fibers in each of these tracts, the kind of information carried, and the side of the body represented.

10. Describe the arterial supply of the spinal cord.

The spinal cord is pretty small, but it's important out of proportion to its size. It's the home of all the motor neurons that work your body, and of a large percentage of the autonomic motor neurons as well. It's also the recipient of nearly all the sensory information taken in by your body. Beyond that, many of the organizing principles of spinal cord reflexes and pathways apply to other parts of the CNS.

1. Posterior and anterior horns of spinal gray matter divide the spinal white matter into funiculi.

The gray matter core of the spinal cord is roughly in the shape of an **H** with a dorsal-ventral orientation at all levels. The dorsally directed limbs of the **H** are the posterior (or dorsal) horns, and the ventrally directed limbs are the anterior (or ventral) horns. The posterior horn, derived from the alar plate of the neural tube, is a sensory processing area that receives most of the afferents that arrive in ipsilateral dorsal roots. The anterior horn is derived from the basal plate and contains the motor neurons whose axons form the ventral roots. At some spinal levels (see section 5 in this chapter) autonomic motor neurons are located in the intermediate zone between the anterior and posterior horns; the axons of these neurons also leave in the ventral roots.

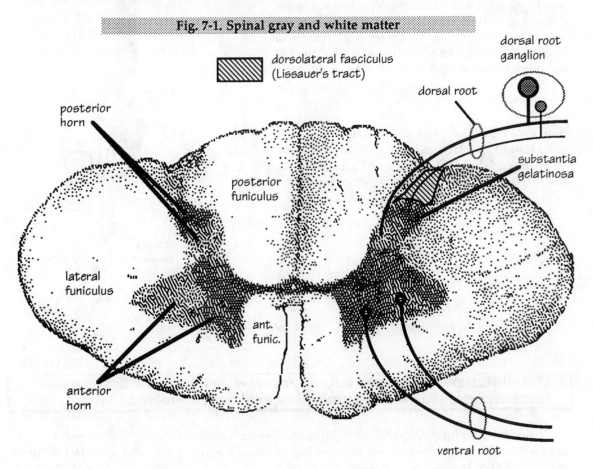

Fig. 7-1. Spinal gray and white matter

dorsolateral fasciculus (Lissauer's tract)

dorsal root ganglion

dorsal root

posterior horn

posterior funiculus

substantia gelatinosa

lateral funiculus

ant. funic.

anterior horn

ventral root

The anterior and posterior horns divide the surrounding spinal white matter into anterior, lateral and posterior funiculi (funiculus means string in Latin).

56

As dorsal roots approach the spinal cord, the afferent fibers are sorted out so that large-diameter fibers enter medial to small-diameter fibers. The large-diameter fibers, carrying touch and position information, either travel rostrally in the posterior funiculus or end in deeper portions of the posterior horn. The small-diameter fibers, primarily carrying pain and temperature information, travel in the dorsolateral fasciculus (Lissauer's tract) to termination sites in a superficial zone of the posterior horn called the substantia gelatinosa.

---

2. The spinal cord contains 8 cervical, 12 thoracic, 5 lumbar, 5 sacral and 1 coccygeal segment.

The spinal cord has a cervical and a lumbar enlargement, serving the needs of the arm and the leg respectively, and ends at the pointed conus medullaris. The conus medullaris is located at *vertebral* level L1/L2, so dorsal and ventral roots from progressively more caudal levels need to travel progressively longer distances through spinal subarachnoid space before reaching their intervertebral foramina of entry or exit. The collection of spinal nerves in subarachnoid space caudal to the conus medullaris is the cauda equina (Latin for horse's tail).

Spinal nerves C1-C7 use the foramen *above* the corresponding vertebra, C8 uses the foramen between vertebrae C7 and T1, and all others use the foramen *below* the corresponding vertebra.

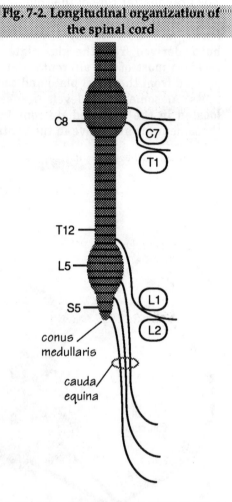

Fig. 7-2. Longitudinal organization of the spinal cord

C8

C7

T1

T12

L5

S5

L1

L2

conus medullaris

cauda equina

---

3. The stretch reflex involves only one synapse, whereas the flexor reflex involves interneurons and multiple spinal cord segments.

Reflexes are involuntary, stereotyped responses to sensory inputs, and every kind of sensory input is involved in reflex circuitry of one or more types. The simplest kind of reflex imaginable involves a sensory fiber and a motor neuron, with a synapse in the CNS connecting the two. This is the circuit underlying the stretch reflex (also called myotatic reflex or deep tendon reflex), by which a muscle contracts in response to being stretched.

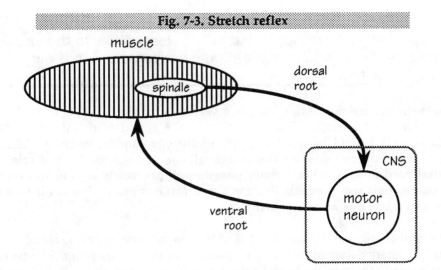

Fig. 7-3. Stretch reflex

Stretch reflexes are the only monosynaptic reflexes. All others involve one or more interneurons. An example is the flexor reflex (or withdrawal reflex), by which a limb is removed from a painful stimulus. This reflex is considerably more complex than a stretch reflex because all the muscles of a limb, and therefore motor neurons in several spinal segments, come into play.

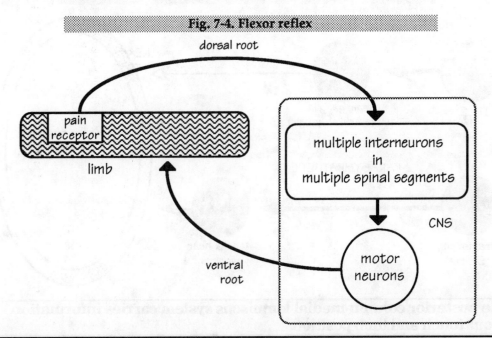

Fig. 7-4. Flexor reflex

4. Motor neurons project directly to skeletal muscle, whereas autonomic control involves a two-neuron chain.

The autonomic nervous system (ANS) does not project efferents from the CNS directly to smooth muscles or glands. Instead, preganglionic autonomic neurons in the CNS project through the ventral roots to postganglionic neurons in ganglia outside the CNS. These postganglionic neurons then project to target organs. (The only exception is the adrenal medulla, which receives autonomic (sympathetic) projections directly from the CNS.) Preganglionic axons are thinly myelinated, while postganglionic axons are unmyelinated.

5. The sympathetic and parasympathetic systems differ in the locations of their preganglionic and postganglionic neurons, and in their postganglionic transmitters.

The sympathetic subdivision of the ANS, in a very general sense the "fight or flight" part of the system, has all its preganglionic neurons in the spinal cord (intermediolateral cell column, forming a lateral horn) at thoracic and upper lumbar levels. (Hence it is also called the thoracolumbar outflow.) The postganglionic neurons are located relatively close to the spinal cord in sympathetic chain ganglia and prevertebral ganglia. Preganglionic sympathetic neurons use acetylcholine for a neurotransmitter. Almost all postganglionic sympathetic neurons use norepinephrine.

The parasympathetic subdivision of the ANS, in a very general sense the energy-absorption and energy-storage part of the system, has some of its preganglionic neurons in the brainstem and others in the sacral spinal cord. (Hence it is also called the craniosacral outflow.) The postganglionic neurons are located in ganglia near or in the target organs. Both preganglionic and postganglionic neurons of the parasympathetic subdivision use acetylcholine for a neurotransmitter.

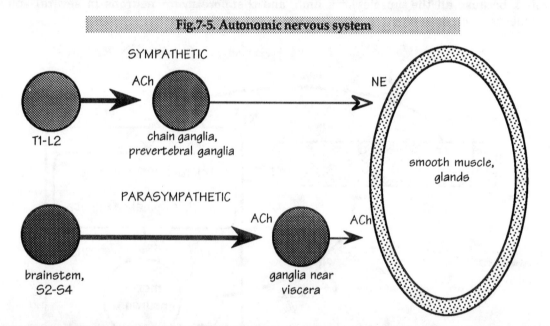

Fig.7-5. Autonomic nervous system

6. The posterior column-medial lemniscus system carries information about touch and limb position.

Most kinds of information travel in more than one pathway in the spinal cord and elsewhere, so damage to a single pathway seldom causes total loss of a function. However, for each function there is usually one pathway that is more important than all the others. In the case of tactile and position sense the most important pathway is the posterior column-medial lemniscus system.

Large-diameter primary afferents, carrying touch and position information, send collaterals through the ipsilateral posterior funiculus. Incoming collaterals add on laterally to those already present in the posterior column, so that by cervical levels the posterior column is subdivided into a medial fasciculus gracilis, representing the leg, and a more lateral fasciculus cuneatus, representing the arm. Fasciculi gracilis and cuneatus then terminate in nuclei gracilis and cuneatus, the posterior column nuclei of the caudal medulla. Second order fibers from neurons of the posterior column nuclei cross the midline and form the medial lemniscus, which ascends through the brainstem to the ventral posterolateral (VPL) nucleus of the thalamus. VPL neurons then project to somatosensory cortex of the postcentral gyrus and adjacent areas.

Fig. 7-6. Posterior column-medial lemniscus pathway

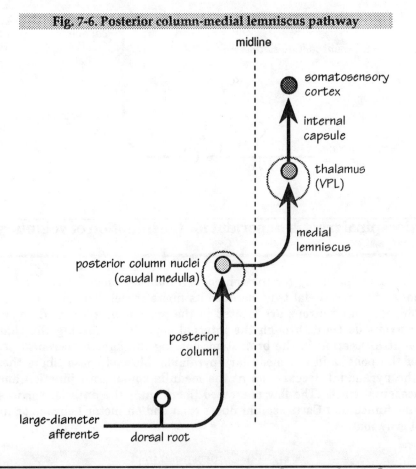

7. The spinothalamic tract carries information about pain and temperature.

The most important pathway for pain and temperature information is the spinothalamic tract; it also carries some touch information. Spinothalamic neurons (i.e., the second-order cells) are located in the spinal cord so this pathway, unlike the posterior column-medial lemniscus pathway, crosses the midline in the spinal cord. Small-diameter primary afferents, carrying pain and temperature and some touch information, traverse the dorsolateral fasciculus (Lissauer's tract) and end on spinothalamic neurons in the posterior horn. Small neurons of the substantia gelatinosa regulate the transmission of information at this synapse. The axons of spinothalamic neurons then cross the midline and form the spinothalamic tract, which ascends through the brainstem to the ventral posterolateral (VPL) nucleus and other nuclei of the thalamus. These thalamic neurons then project to somatosensory cortex of the postcentral gyrus and adjacent areas.

60

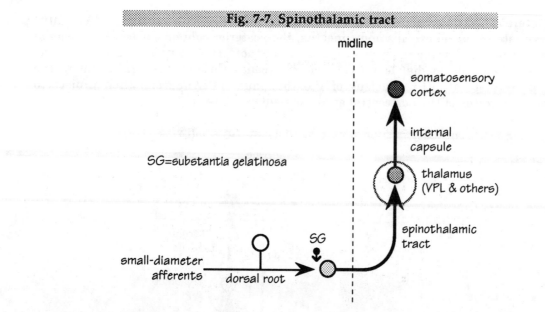

Fig. 7-7. Spinothalamic tract

SG=substantia gelatinosa

somatosensory cortex

internal capsule

thalamus (VPL & others)

spinothalamic tract

small-diameter afferents

dorsal root

SG

8. The corticospinal tract is important for the initiation of voluntary movement.

The most important pathway for the control of voluntary movement is the corticospinal tract (also called the pyramidal tract because its fibers travel through the pyramids of the medulla). Corticospinal neurons are located in the precentral gyrus and adjacent cortical areas. Their axons descend through the internal capsule (bypassing the thalamus) and travel in a ventral location in the brainstem, passing through the cerebral peduncle, the basal part of the pons, and the medullary pyramids. Most of these fibers then cross the midline in the pyramidal decussation at the medulla-spinal cord junction and enter the lateral corticospinal tract. (The few uncrossed fibers enter the anterior corticospinal tract in the anterior funiculus.) Corticospinal fibers then end on motor neurons or interneurons of the spinal gray matter.

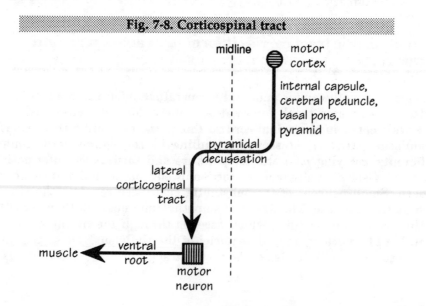

Fig. 7-8. Corticospinal tract

midline

motor cortex

internal capsule, cerebral peduncle, basal pons, pyramid

pyramidal decussation

lateral corticospinal tract

muscle

ventral root

motor neuron

9. Axons with similar functions are grouped into tracts in the spinal cord.

Fig. 7-9. Major spinal cord tracts

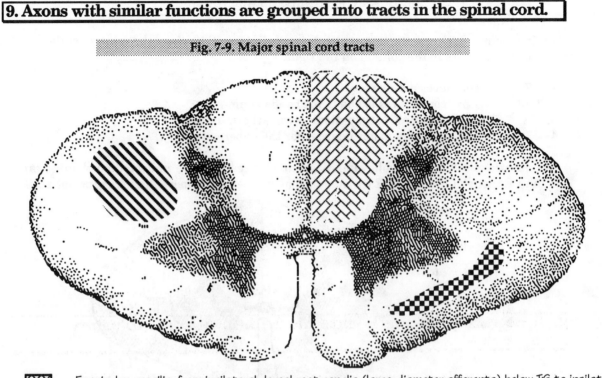

 Fasciculus gracilis: from ipsilateral dorsal root ganglia (large-diameter afferents) below T6 to ipsilatera nucleus gracilis; touch and some position information from ipsilateral leg.

 Fasciculus cuneatus: from ipsilateral dorsal root ganglia (large-diameter afferents) above T6 to ipsilateral nucleus cuneatus; touch and position information from ipsilateral arm.

 Spinothalamic tract: from contralateral posterior horn to thalamus; pain and temperature and some touch information from contralateral half of body.

 Lateral corticospinal tract: from contralateral motor cortex to motor neurons and interneurons; principal pathway for voluntary movement.

10. Anterior and posterior spinal arteries supply the spinal cord.

Each vertebral artery gives rise to an anterior and a posterior spinal artery. The posterior spinal arteries form a plexiform network that travels along the line of attachment of the dorsal roots and supplies the posterior columns, the posterior horns, and part of the lateral corticospinal tract. The two anterior spinal arteries fuse and travel along the midline of the spinal cord, supplying its anterior two thirds. Both anterior and posterior spinal arteries receive blood from segmental arteries at various levels, so that blood from the vertebral artery only reaches cervical segments.

62

Self-Evaluation Questions

For questions 1-4, choose the best match between the spinal levels in the column on the left and the contents in the column on the right.

1. C7
2. C10
3. T2
4. S3

a) does not exist
b) contributes axons to the cauda equina
c) contains preganglionic sympathetic neurons
d) contains motor neurons for the upper extremity

For questions 5-8, use the following diagram. Choices A–D are indicated on the diagram, and E=none of the above. Each answer may be used once, more than once, or not at all.

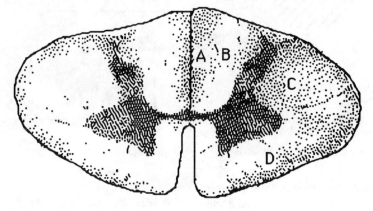

5. Arise from cell bodies in the contralateral posterior horn.
6. Collaterals of these fibers participate in the triceps stretch reflex.
7. These fibers have their cell bodies in contralateral dorsal root ganglia below T6.
8. Some of these fibers arise in the contralateral precentral gyrus.

9. The neural circuitry of the stretch reflex involves
a) multiple interneurons in multiple spinal cord segments.
b) small-diameter primary afferents.
c) Golgi tendon organs.
d both (a) and (c)
e) none of the above

10. Sympathetic motor neurons in the spinal cord
a) have axons that end directly on smooth muscles and glands.
b) have axons that end in ganglia near or within smooth muscles and glands.
c) are typically involved in "fight or flight" types of activities.
d) none of the above

11. A distinctive neurological disease called syringomyelia involves cavitation and enlargement of the central canal, typically of the lower cervical cord, at the expense of surrounding neural tissues. What do you think would be the first neurological symptoms of such a process? What would happen next?

12. Loss of deep tendon reflexes can result from damage to either the afferent or the efferent portion of the reflex arc. How could you determine whether a patient with hypoactive reflexes in part of the body had suffered damage to dorsal or ventral roots?

13. A left-handed, 42-year-old, male professional beer drinker awoke one morning, following a strenuous workout with his team, with generalized weakness in the upper and lower extremities of both sides and pronounced bilateral diminution of pain and temperature sensibility on both sides of the body below the neck. There was no apparent disturbance of position sense, vibratory sensibility, or tactile discrimination. Can you localize the problem anatomically?

Answers and Explanations

1. **d**. Part of the cervical enlargment.

2. **a**. There are only 8 cervical segments.

3. **c**.

4. **b**. See Fig. 7-2 (or text Fig. 7-2B–D, p. 122).

5. **d**. Spinothalamic tract.

6. **b**. Fasciculus cuneatus, large-diameter primary afferents from the upper extremity.

7. **e**. Primary afferents usually don't cross the midline.

8. **c**. Corticospinal tract.

9. **e**. See Fig. 7-3.

10. **c**. See Section 5 in this chapter.

11. The first thing to go would be the fibers crossing in the anterior white commissure to form the spinothalamic tracts of both sides at that level. This would lead to loss of pain and temperature sensation bilaterally in the dermatomes represented in the damaged segments (dermatomes would correspond to spinal levels 1-2 segments caudal to the actual damage; see text Fig. 7-17, p. 139). Subsequent damage is variable, but typically involves nearby lower motor neurons, causing weakness and eventually atrophy of muscles innervated by affected segments.

12. Segments affected can be determined on the basis of the reflexes affected. Then the appropriate dermatomes can be tested for sensory loss. Also, ventral root damage eventually results in muscle atrophy, while dorsal root damage does not. Perhaps most simply, the patient will still be able to contract the muscle voluntarily if its afferent innervation is defective, even though reflexes involving the muscle may be hypoactive.

13. Weakness of all extremities suggests bilateral damage to lateral corticospinal tracts. Bilateral diminution of pain and temperature sensation suggests damage to lateral spinothalamic tracts on both sides. Together these findings imply damage to both lateral funiculi. Intact tactile sensibility implies intact posterior columns. The anterior spinal artery (see text Fig. 7-26, p. 150) supplies the entire cord except for the posterior horns and columns, and its occlusion could produce such damage extending over one or a few segments. Supply of the lateral corticospinal tract may be partially from the posterior spinal artery, so the degree of weakness is variable from one case to another. This is the classic anterior spinal artery syndrome.

CHAPTER 8

BRAINSTEM

LEARNING OBJECTIVES

1. List the attachment points and the general functions of cranial nerves III-XII.

2. Indicate the locations of the following surface features of the brainstem: superior and inferior colliculi, cerebral peduncle, basal part of the pons, middle cerebellar peduncle, pyramid and olive.

3. Describe the major characteristic features of each the following brainstem levels, as seen in cross section: caudal medulla, rostral medulla, caudal pons, rostral pons, caudal midbrain and rostral midbrain. Indicate the location of the medial lemniscus, spinothalamic tract and corticospinal tract at each of these levels.

4. Indicate the location of the brainstem reticular formation, and indicate in a general sense its role in the control of sensory functions, motor functions, and consciousness.

The brainstem is another part of the CNS whose importance is out of proportion to its size. It does the same basic sensory and motor functions for the head that the spinal cord does for the body, and it takes care of some special senses as well (hearing, equilibrium, taste). It also contains a reticular core whose activity is crucial for the maintenance of consciousness.

1. Cranial nerves III-XII are attached to the midbrain, pons and medulla.

The olfactory nerve (I) is a series of thin filaments that attach directly to the olfactory bulb, part of the telencephalon. Fibers of the optic nerve (II) proceed through the the optic chiasm and tract, and most end in the lateral geniculate nucleus of the thalamus, part of the diencephalon. The ten remaining cranial nerves originate or terminate in the brainstem, as indicated in the following table; V, L and D indicate that the attachment points are located on the ventral, lateral or dorsal surface of the brainstem. Text Fig. 8-3, pp. 156–157, shows photographs of all these attachment points.

Cranial Nerve	Main Functions	Attachment Point
III. Oculomotor	eye movements, pupil, lens	rostral midbrain (V)
IV. Trochlear	eye movements	pons/midbrain junction (D)
V. Trigeminal	facial sensation, chewing	midpons (L)
VI. Abducens	eye movements	pontomedullary junction (V)
VII. Facial	taste, facial expression	pontomedullary junction (V/L)
VIII. Vestibulocochlear	hearing, equilibrium	pontomedullary junction (V/L)
IX. Glossopharyngeal	taste, swallowing	rostral medulla (L)
X. Vagus	visceral sensory and motor; speaking, swallowing	rostral medulla (L)
XI. Accessory*	head and shoulder movements	caudal medulla, upper cervical spinal cord (L)
XII. Hypoglossal	tongue movements	rostral medulla (V/L)

*Some of the motor axons that travel with the vagus to throat muscles are often considered
  separately as a cranial branch of the accessory nerve.

At its attachment point, each of these cranial nerves is carrying sensory information from ipsilateral receptors or motor output to ipsilateral muscles (except for the case of visceral afferents and efferents, where the ipsilateral-contralateral concept loses much of its meaning). Thus, the right vestibulocochlear nerve carries information from the right cochlea and the left oculomotor nerve innervates muscles of the left eye. Similarly, the fibers of these cranial nerves mostly terminate in or originate from the ipsilateral side of the CNS. The principal exceptions are the trochlear and oculomotor nerves. All trochlear fibers and some oculomotor fibers originate from motor neurons in the contralateral half of the CNS.

2. Different surface features characterize different rostral-caudal levels of the brainstem.

Various nuclei and fiber bundles form surface features at different levels of the brainstem. The most prominent of these are listed in this section; photographs can be seen in text Fig. 8-3, pp. 156–157.

Midbrain

Superior colliculi, two rounded elevations on the dorsal surface of the rostral midbrain, involved in eye movements and the direction of visual attention; inferior colliculi, two rounded elevations on the dorsal surface of the caudal midbrain, part of the auditory pathway; cerebral peduncles, large paired fiber bundles on the ventral surface of the midbrain, each carrying the corticospinal, corticobulbar and corticopontine tracts.

Pons

Basal part of the pons, a large transverse band of fibers and nuclei for which the pons is named (pons is Latin for bridge), the nuclei of each side receiving inputs via the ipsilateral corticopontine tract; middle cerebellar peduncles, fibers on each side of the pons that originated in contralateral pontine nuclei, passed transversely in the basal part of the pons, and are now moving into ipsilateral cerebellar cortex.

Medulla

Pyramids, paired longitudinal bundles of fibers on the ventral surface of the medulla, made up of the corticospinal tracts; olive, an ovoid bump dorsolateral to each pyramid in the rostral medulla and underlain by the inferior olivary nucleus, an important component of cerebellar circuitry.

---

3. The nuclei and tracts underlying surface elevations, together with other features, characterize different levels of the brainstem.

The medulla, pons and midbrain are commonly divided into rostral and caudal halves using some of the surface elevations described above and some other features. Each of these six brainstem levels has a few major, characteristic structures. Also, at each of these levels the corticospinal tract is in a ventral location and the medial lemniscus is medial to the spinothalamic tract.

The caudal or closed medulla is the part that does not contain any of the fourth ventricle; it extends from the pyramidal decussation to the beginning of the fourth ventricle. The rostral or open medulla is the part that contains a portion of the fourth ventricle; it extends from the caudal end of the fourth ventricle to the point at which the brainstem becomes attached to the cerebellum by the inferior and middle cerebellar peduncles. All of the pons contains part of the fourth ventricle; the caudal pons is the part physically attached to the cerebellum, primarily by the middle cerebellar peduncle. The rostral pons is no longer connected to the cerebellum; the trigeminal nerve is attached to the brainstem at the caudal pons-rostral pons junction. The midbrain encloses the cerebral aqueduct; the caudal midbrain is the part containing the inferior colliculi, the rostral midbrain the part containing the superior colliculi. The trochlear nerve emerges at the pons-midbrain junction, and the posterior commissure is located at the midbrain-diencephalon junction.

The following figures indicate the major features of each of these brainstem levels. Information about the functions and connections of each can be found in the text and in Chapters 9A-C of this Study Guide; some of the structures have not been mentioned yet and may not make sense until you have read Chapters 9A-C.

67

Fig. 8-1. Caudal medulla

Caudal Medulla
(compare to text Fig. 9-41,
pp. 224–225)

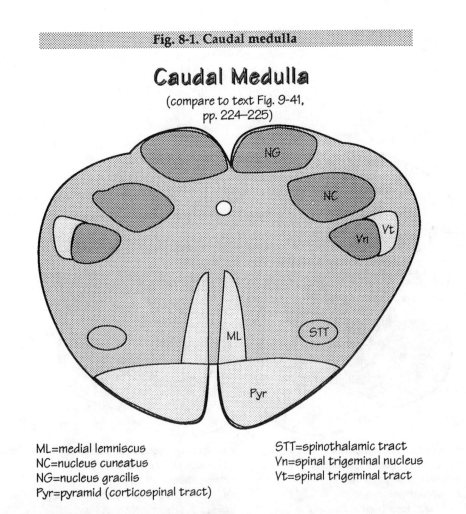

ML=medial lemniscus
NC=nucleus cuneatus
NG=nucleus gracilis
Pyr=pyramid (corticospinal tract)

STT=spinothalamic tract
Vn=spinal trigeminal nucleus
Vt=spinal trigeminal tract

Other important features of the caudal medulla
The posterior columns (fasciculi gracilis and cuneatus) terminate in the posterior column nuclei (nuclei gracilis and cuneatus). Second order fibers from the posterior column nuclei cross the midline and form the medial lemniscus.
Most corticospinal tract fibers cross in the pyramidal decussation (at the spinomedullary junction) to form the lateral corticospinal tract.
Trigeminal pain and temperature fibers, traveling through the spinal trigeminal tract, end in the spinal trigeminal nucleus (see Chapter 9B).

Fig. 8-2. Rostral medulla

Rostral Medulla

(compare to text Fig. 9-42,
pp. 226–227)

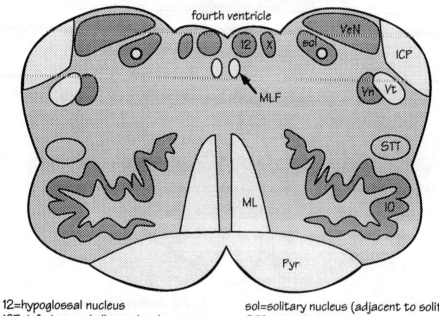

12=hypoglossal nucleus
ICP=inferior cerebellar peduncle
IO=inferior olivary nucleus
ML=medial lemniscus
MLF=medial longitudinal fasciculus
Pyr=pyramid (corticospinal tract)

sol=solitary nucleus (adjacent to solitary tract)
STT=spinothalamic tract
VeN=vestibular nuclei
Vn=spinal trigeminal nucleus
Vt=spinal trigeminal tract
X=dorsal motor nucleus of the vagus

Other important features of the rostral medulla

Olivocerebellar fibers cross the midline and form the bulk of the inferior cerebellar peduncle.

Nucleus ambiguus (➛cranial nerves IX and X).

Cochlear nuclei at the pontomedullary junction.

Caudal Pons

(compare to text Fig. 9-44,
pp. 230–231)

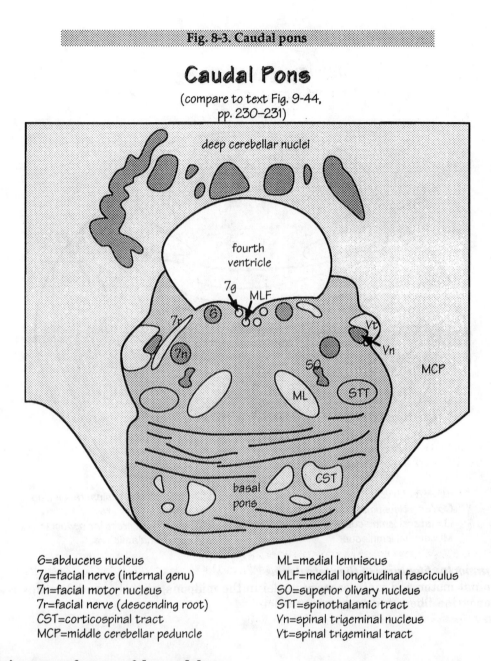

6=abducens nucleus
7g=facial nerve (internal genu)
7n=facial motor nucleus
7r=facial nerve (descending root)
CST=corticospinal tract
MCP=middle cerebellar peduncle

ML=medial lemniscus
MLF=medial longitudinal fasciculus
SO=superior olivary nucleus
STT=spinothalamic tract
Vn=spinal trigeminal nucleus
Vt=spinal trigeminal tract

Other important features of the caudal pons
Cochlear nuclei at the pontomedullary junction.
Trapezoid body and the beginning of the lateral lemniscus.
Internal genu of the facial nerve.
Corticopontine fibers end in pontine nuclei.
Superior cerebellar peduncle begins to emerge from the deep cerebellar nuclei.
Trigeminal motor and main sensory nuclei in the midpons, slightly rostral to this level.

Fig. 8-4. Rostral pons

Rostral Pons

(compare to text Fig. 9-46,
pp. 236–237)

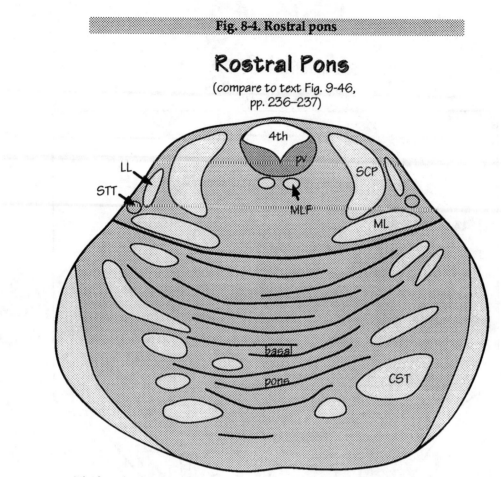

4th=fourth ventricle
CST=corticospinal tract
LL=lateral lemniscus
ML=medial lemniscus

MLF=medial longitudinal fasciculus
pv=periventricular gray
SCP=superior cerebellar peduncle
STT=spinothalamic tract

Other important features of the rostral pons

Trigeminal motor and main sensory nuclei in the midpons, slightly caudal to this level.
Corticopontine fibers end in pontine nuclei.

Fig. 8-5. Caudal midbrain

Caudal Midbrain

(compare to text Fig. 9-47,
pp. 238–239)

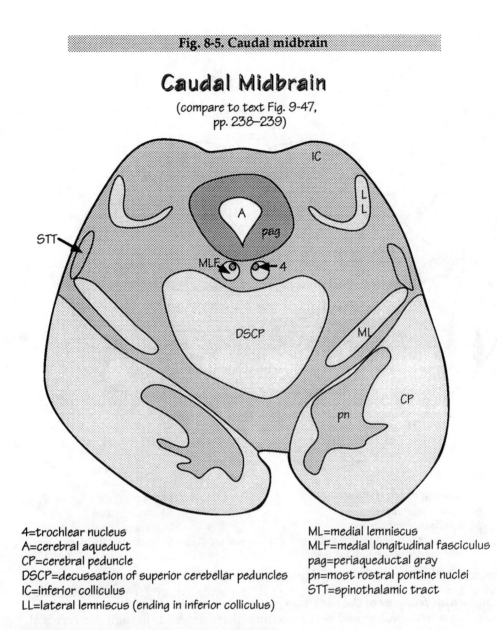

4=trochlear nucleus
A=cerebral aqueduct
CP=cerebral peduncle
DSCP=decussation of superior cerebellar peduncles
IC=inferior colliculus
LL=lateral lemniscus (ending in inferior colliculus)

ML=medial lemniscus
MLF=medial longitudinal fasciculus
pag=periaqueductal gray
pn=most rostral pontine nuclei
STT=spinothalamic tract

Other important features of the caudal midbrain

Corticospinal, corticobulbar and corticopontine fibers descend through the cerebral peduncle.

Lateral lemniscus ends in the inferior colliculus, inferior brachium emerges from the inferior colliculus.

Fig. 8-6. Rostral midbrain

Rostral Midbrain

(compare to text Fig. 9-48,
pp. 240–241)

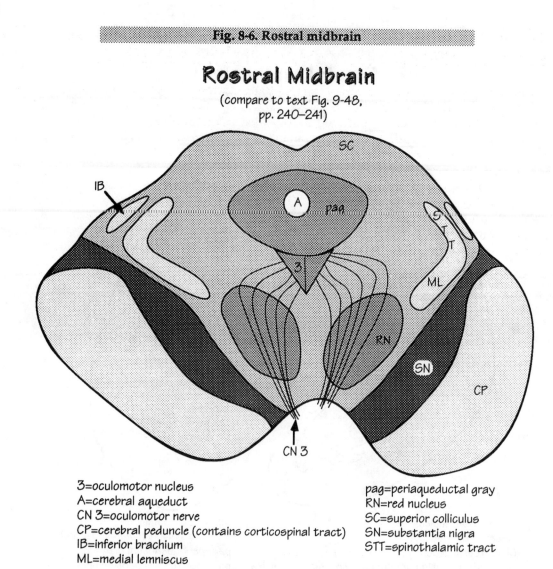

3=oculomotor nucleus
A=cerebral aqueduct
CN 3=oculomotor nerve
CP=cerebral peduncle (contains corticospinal tract)
IB=inferior brachium
ML=medial lemniscus

pag=periaqueductal gray
RN=red nucleus
SC=superior colliculus
SN=substantia nigra
STT=spinothalamic tract

Other important features of the rostral midbrain

Corticospinal, corticobulbar and corticopontine fibers descend through the cerebral peduncle.

Crossed fibers of the superior cerebellar peduncles pass through or around the red nucleus; some terminate in the red nucleus.

Inferior brachium begins to terminate in the medial geniculate nucleus of the thalamus.

Optic tract fibers reach the superior colliculus via the superior brachium.

4. The brainstem reticular formation exerts some control over sensory, motor and visceral functions, and over our level of consciousness as well.

The reticular formation forms a core of neural tissue in the brainstem, surrounded by the major nuclei and tracts mentioned thus far. It samples the information carried by most sensory, motor and visceral pathways. The reticular formation uses some of this information in various reflexes (e.g., circulatory and respiratory reflexes, swallowing, coughing). It also sends outputs caudally to the spinal cord and rostrally to the diencephalon. The outputs to the spinal cord mediate some aspects of movement, control the sensitivity of spinal reflexes, and regulate the transmission of sensory information (especially pain) into ascending pathways. The outputs to the diencephalon from a portion of the reticular formation called the Ascending Reticular Activating System (ARAS) modulate the level of cortical activity and hence the level of consciousness; the ARAS is important in sleep-wakefulness cycles.

Self-Evaluation Questions

For questions 1–5, match the cranial nerves in the column on the left with the properties in the column on the right; a given property may be used more than once or not at all.

1. Cranial nerve IV
2. Cranial nerve V
3. Cranial nerve VII
4. Cranial nerve X
5. Cranial nerve XII

a) motor nerve for muscles of facial expression
b) attached to the dorsal surface of the brainstem
c) controls the size of the pupil
d) attached to the brainstem at a midpons level
e) visceral sensory and motor functions
f) controls tongue muscles

For questions 6–10, choose the best match between the brainstem levels in the column on the left and the structures in the column on the right.

6. caudal medulla
7. rostral medulla
8. caudal pons
9. caudal midbrain
10. rostral midbrain

a) red nucleus
b) trapezoid body
c) nucleus gracilis
d) inferior olivary nucleus
e) decussation of superior cerebellar peduncles

74

1. **b.**

2. **d.**

3. **a.**

4. **e.**

5. **f.**

6. **c.**

7. **d.**

8. **b.**

9. **e.**

10. **a.**

CHAPTER 9A

OCULOMOTOR, TROCHLEAR, ABDUCENS AND HYPOGLOSSAL NERVES

LEARNING OBJECTIVES

1. List the contents of the nuclei of the oculomotor, trochlear, abducens and hypoglossal nerves.

2. Indicate the locations within the brainstem of the nuclei of the oculomotor, trochlear, abducens and hypoglossal nuclei.

3. Specify the functions of the two cell types found in the abducens nucleus. Indicate the role of the paramedian pontine reticular formation and the medial longitudinal fasciculus in horizontal eye movements.

4. Differentiate between the effects of damage to the hypoglossal nerve or nucleus and damage to the corticobulbar fibers to the hypoglossal nucleus.

The oculomotor, trochlear, abducens and hypoglossal nerves are the simplest cranial nerves, in the sense that they just contain motor axons to ordinary skeletal muscle (except for some clinically important autonomics in the oculomotor nerve). Their nuclei are near the midline, as expected from the embryological development of the brainstem.

1. The oculomotor, trochlear, abducens and hypoglossal nuclei control eye movements and tongue movements.

The trochlear nerve (IV) innervates the superior oblique muscle and the abducens nerve (VI) innervates the lateral rectus. The oculomotor nerve (III) innervates the remaining extraocular muscles (medial, superior and inferior recti, inferior oblique) and the levator of the eyelid, and also contains the preganglionic parasympathetic fibers for the pupillary sphincter and the ciliary muscle. All three of these nerves, once they leave the brainstem, proceed to the ipsilateral eye (although trochlear and some oculomotor fibers cross before leaving the brainstem).

The hypoglossal nerve (XII) innervates the muscles of the ipsilateral half of the tongue.

2. The oculomotor, trochlear, abducens and hypoglossal nuclei are located near the midline of the brainstem in the floor of the ventricular system.

As expected from their embryological development, the oculomotor, trochlear, abducens and hypoglossal nuclei are located near the midline in the floor of the ventricular system. The oculomotor nucleus is in the rostral midbrain (text Fig. 9-3, p. 181), the trochlear nucleus in the caudal midbrain (text Fig. 9-4, p. 182), the abducens nucleus in the caudal pons (text Fig. 9-5B, p. 183) and the hypoglossal nucleus in the rostral medulla (text Fig. 9-10, p. 187).

3. The abducens nucleus contains not only lateral rectus motor neurons, but also interneurons that project through the MLF to the contralateral oculomotor nucleus.

Any time we look to the left or the right, we need to simultaneously contract the lateral rectus of one eye and the medial rectus of the other eye. Theoretically, this could be accomplished by having separate, parallel inputs to both sets of motor neurons. However, we have evolved a different mechanism to accomplish the same end. The abducens nucleus contains not only the motor neurons for the ipsilateral lateral rectus, but also an equal number of interneurons whose axons cross the midline, join the medial longitudinal fasciculus (MLF) and ascend to medial rectus motor neurons in the contralateral oculomotor nucleus. All excitatory inputs to the abducens nucleus end on both motor neurons and interneurons, so coordinated gaze is achieved every time we try to contract one lateral rectus.

Inputs to the abducens nucleus arise in a number of sites, including the vestibular nuclei (this allows us to generate eye movements equal and opposite to head movements—the vestibuloocular reflex). Ordinary voluntary eye movements are of a rapid type called saccades. Making a rapid eye movement over to a target requires a rapid initial burst of action potentials in abducens motor neurons and interneurons to get the eyes moving, followed by slower maintained firing to maintain the new position. The required timing signals are generated in the reticular formation near the abducens nucleus, a region called the paramedian pontine reticular formation (or PPRF, or pontine gaze center).

Hence, damage to one abducens nucleus causes loss of *all* horizontal eye movements to the ipsilateral side, but damage to the PPRF causes selective loss of rapid eye movements to the ipsilateral side. (Eye movements are discussed more fully in Chapter 12.)

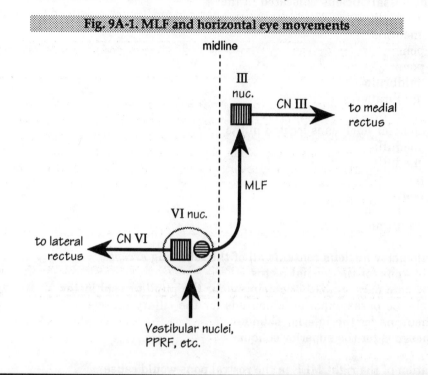

Fig. 9A-1. MLF and horizontal eye movements

4. Weakness of one side of the tongue causes it to deviate to that side.

A normal tongue when protruded stays in the midline, in part because the muscles of each side of the tongue push toward the midline with equal force. Hence, if one side of the tongue is weak the normal side will push the tongue past the midline and it will deviate *toward* the weak side. In the case of damage to the hypoglossal nerve or nucleus the weakness is accompanied by fasciculations and atrophy, typical signs of lower motor neuron damage.

Upper motor neurons for tongue motor neurons, like those for spinal cord motor neurons, are located in the precentral gyrus and adjacent cortical areas. Their axons, called corticobulbar fibers, accompany corticospinal axons through the internal capsule, cerebral peduncle and pons. In the rostral medulla, they leave the corticospinal fibers and innervate the hypoglossal nucleus. As they do so, many but not all of them cross the midline. Hence both sides of the tongue can be made to contract by one cerebral hemisphere, and unilateral damage to corticobulbar fibers does not cause profound weakness of one side of the tongue. If, however, in a given individual there are substantially more crossed than uncrossed fibers, then there may be some transient weakness on the contralateral side following corticobulbar damage. In such an individual, cortical damage would cause tongue deviation *away* from the side of the lesion, since the weak side would be contralateral to the lesion.

Self-Evaluation Questions

1. The hypoglossal nucleus is located in the
   a) caudal medulla
   b) rostral medulla
   c) caudal pons
   d) rostral pons
   e) caudal midbrain
   f) rostral midbrain

2. The oculomotor nucleus is located in the
   a) caudal medulla
   b) rostral medulla
   c) caudal pons
   d) rostral pons
   e) caudal midbrain
   f) rostral midbrain

3. The oculomotor nucleus contains all of the following *except*
   a) motor neurons for the medial rectus
   b) preganglionic parasympathetic neurons for the pupillary sphincter
   c) preganglionic parasympathetic neurons for the ciliary muscle
   d) motor neurons for the inferior oblique
   e) motor neurons for the superior oblique

4. Stimulation of the right MLF in the rostral pons would cause
   a) both eyes to move to the left.
   b) both eyes to move to the right.
   c) the left eye to move to the left.
   d) the left eye to move to the right.
   e) the right eye to move to the left.
   f) the right eye to move to the right.

5. The paramedian pontine reticular formation produces the timing signals for
   a) rapid eye movements to the ipsilateral side.
   b) rapid eye movements to the contralateral side.
   c) all eye movements to the ipsilateral side.
   d) all eye movements to the contralateral side.

6. Damage to motor cortex on one side would cause the tongue, when protruded, to deviate to
   a) the side of the damage.
   b) the side opposite the damage.

7. The oculomotor, trochlear, abducens and hypoglossal nuclei all
   a) contain approximately equal numbers of motor neurons and interneurons.
   b) contain appreciable numbers of motor neurons whose axons cross the midline before leaving the brainstem.
   c) are located near the midline and in or near the floor of the ventricular system.
   d) contain both motor neurons and preganglionic parasympathetic neurons.

Answers and Explanations

1. **b.**

2. **f.**

3. **e.** These are in the trochlear nucleus.

4. **e.** These fibers are on their way to ipsilateral medial rectus motor neurons.

5. **a.** All horizontal eye movements use the abducens interneurons and MLF, but only rapid eye movements use the timing signals generated in the PPRF.

6. **b.** The side opposite the damage is slightly weak, and the tongue deviates toward the weak side.

7. **c.** Location near the midline is expected from embryology (see text Fig. 9-1, p.177). Only the abducens nucleus has large numbers of interneurons; no abducens motor neurons have crossed projections; of these three, only the oculomotor nucleus contains preganglionic parasympathetics.

CHAPTER 9B

TRIGEMINAL, FACIAL, GLOSSOPHARYNGEAL, VAGAL AND ACCESSORY NERVES

LEARNING OBJECTIVES

1. List the contents of the trigeminal nerve, and indicate the location within the brainstem of the nuclei associated with the trigeminal nerve.

2. Diagram the central pathways by which information from the head about touch, pain and temperature reach consciousness.

3. Describe the somatotopic arrangement of fibers and their terminations in the spinal tract and nucleus of the trigeminal nerve.

4. Indicate the location within the brainstem of the facial motor nucleus, and describe the course taken by facial nerve fibers after they leave this nucleus. Differentiate between the effects of damage to the facial nerve or nucleus and damage to the corticobulbar fibers to the facial nucleus.

5. Indicate the location within the brainstem of motor neurons for the larynx and pharynx, and the cranial nerves through which these motor neurons distribute their axons. Differentiate between the effects of damage to the nerves or nucleus and damage to the corticobulbar fibers to the nucleus.

6. Indicate the location within the brainstem of preganglionic parasympathetic neurons, and the cranial nerves through which these neurons distribute their axons.

7. List the cranial nerves through which visceral afferent information reaches the brainstem. Indicate where these afferents travel within the brainstem and where they terminate.

8. List the cranial nerves through which information from taste buds reaches the brainstem. Diagram the route through which this gustatory information reaches consciousness.

9. Diagram the neural circuitry involved in the jaw-jerk and blink reflexes.

The trigeminal, facial, glossopharyngeal, vagus and accessory nerves are more complex than the ones considered in the last chapter. Each innervates skeletal muscle derived embryologically from the branchial arches. Except for the accessory nerve, each has more than one kind of fiber. Nevertheless, each has only one or two major functions (see the table at the beginning of Chapter 8).

1. The trigeminal is the somatic sensory nerve for the head and the motor nerve for chewing.

The trigeminal nerve (V) is the principal somatosensory nerve for the head. The afferent fibers have cell bodies in the trigeminal ganglion (except for a few, mainly from muscle spindles, whose cell bodies are *inside* the CNS in the mesencephalic nucleus of the trigeminal nerve, located in the rostral pons and caudal midbrain). Central processes of these afferent fibers end either in the main sensory nucleus, located in the midpons, or in the spinal trigeminal nucleus, which merges rostrally with the main sensory nucleus and caudally with the posterior horn of the upper cervical spinal cord. The latter fibers reach the spinal trigeminal nucleus by travelling through the spinal trigeminal tract.

Motor neurons for the masseter and several smaller muscles are located in the trigeminal motor nucleus, ventromedial to the main sensory nucleus in the midpons.

2. The trigeminal nerve is involved in pathways analogous to the posterior column system and the spinothalamic tract.

Large-diameter trigeminal afferents, carrying information about touch and jaw position, end in the main sensory nucleus (Fig. 9B-1). The main sensory nucleus is the trigeminal equivalent of a posterior column nucleus. Second order fibers from the main sensory nucleus cross the midline and ascend near the medial lemniscus as part of the ventral trigeminal tract to reach the ventral posteromedial nucleus (VPM) of the thalamus. VPM neurons then project to somatosensory cortex of the postcentral gyrus and adjacent areas. In contrast to the situation in the spinal cord, large-diameter trigeminal afferents do not travel through anything analogous to the posterior columns before reaching their nucleus of termination.

Small-diameter trigeminal afferents, carrying pain and temperature and some touch information, turn caudally in the spinal trigeminal tract. The pain and temperature fibers end in portions of the spinal trigeminal nucleus in the caudal medulla and upper cervical spinal cord (Fig. 9B-1). Second order fibers from the spinal trigeminal nucleus then cross the midline and ascend near the spinothalamic tract as a second part of the ventral trigeminal tract to reach VPM and other thalamic nuclei. Thalamic neurons then project to somatosensory cortex of the postcentral gyrus and adjacent areas. In contrast to the situation in the spinal cord, small-diameter trigeminal afferents travel an appreciable distance (in the spinal trigeminal tract) in the CNS before reaching the second-order neurons on which they terminate.

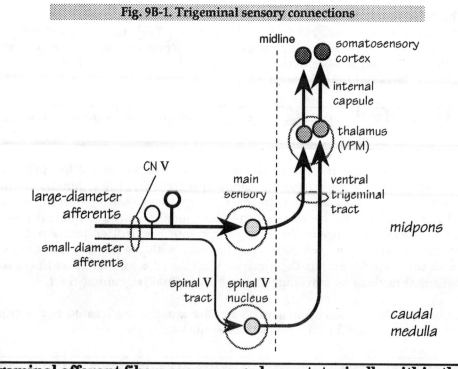

Fig. 9B-1. Trigeminal sensory connections

somatosensory cortex

midline

internal capsule

thalamus (VPM)

CN V

main sensory

ventral trigeminal tract

large-diameter afferents

midpons

small-diameter afferents

spinal V tract | spinal V nucleus

caudal medulla

3. Trigeminal afferent fibers are arranged somatotopically within the brainstem.

The primary afferent fibers in the spinal trigeminal tract are arranged somatotopically, with the ipsilateral half of the face represented upside down (i.e., ophthalmic division fibers most ventral, mandibular division fibers most dorsal). In addition to this dorsal-ventral gradient, there is a rostral-caudal order in which the pain and temperature fibers terminate in the spinal trigeminal nucleus. Fibers representing areas near the midline terminate most rostrally (i.e., in the mid-medulla), and fibers representing areas toward the back of the head terminate most caudally (i.e., in the upper cervical spinal cord). This makes sense, since it means that pain and temperature afferents from the back of the head (i.e., upper cervical roots) end near the termination sites of trigeminal afferents from nearby areas of the head.

4. Facial nerve fibers hook around the abducens nucleus before leaving the brainstem to control the muscles of facial expression.

A major component of the facial nerve (VII) is the axons of the motor neurons for the muscles of facial expression (and the stapedius). These originate in the facial motor nucleus of the caudal pons, but loop around the abducens nucleus as the internal genu of the facial nerve before leaving the brainstem to innervate the ipsilateral half of the face (text Fig. 9-6, p. 184).

Corticobulbar fibers to the motor neurons for the lower half of the face are mostly crossed. However, corticobulbar fibers to the motor neurons for the upper half of the face are distributed bilaterally. Hence, all parts of the face except the ipsilateral lower quadrant can be made to contract by one cerebral hemisphere, and so unilateral corticobulbar damage causes weakness of only the contralateral lower quadrant. (For example, after left motor cortex damage the intact right hemisphere cannot make the muscles of the right lower quadrant contract.) In contrast, unilateral damage to the facial nerve or nucleus causes weakness of the entire *ipsilateral* half of the face.

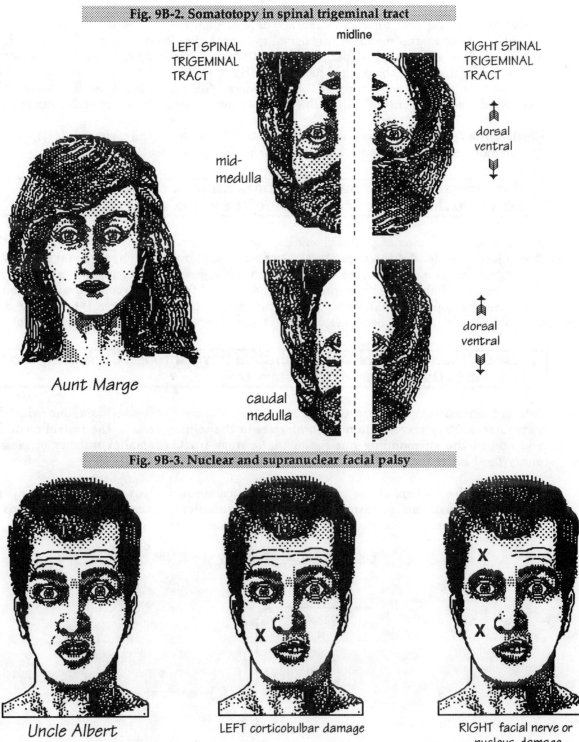

Fig. 9B-2. Somatotopy in spinal trigeminal tract

LEFT SPINAL TRIGEMINAL TRACT

RIGHT SPINAL TRIGEMINAL TRACT

midline

dorsal
ventral

mid-medulla

dorsal
ventral

caudal medulla

Aunt Marge

Fig. 9B-3. Nuclear and supranuclear facial palsy

Uncle Albert

LEFT corticobulbar damage

RIGHT facial nerve or nucleus damage

84

5. Motor neurons for the larynx and pharynx are located in the medulla and have axons that travel with the vagal and glossopharyngeal nerves.

Motor neurons for the muscles of the larynx and pharynx are located in the reticular formation of the rostral medulla, just dorsal to the inferior olivary nucleus, as the nucleus ambiguus. Most of them travel peripherally in the vagus nerve (X) to ipsilateral muscles; a few travel in the glossopharyngeal nerve (IX). (Some of the vagal fibers travel for a short distance with the accessory nerve (XI) before joining the vagus; the latter fibers are often considered a separate cranial part of the accessory nerve rather than part of the vagus.)

Corticobulbar fibers to nucleus ambiguus are distributed bilaterally, so unilateral corticobulbar damage causes no serious laryngeal or pharyngeal deficits.

6. Most preganglionic parasympathetic neurons in the brainstem are located in the dorsal motor nucleus of the vagus.

The principal collection of preganglionic parasympathetic neurons in the brainstem is the dorsal motor nucleus of the vagus nerve, located just lateral to the hypoglossal nucleus in the rostral medulla. Their axons travel through the vagus nerve to ganglia that innervate the thoracic and abdominal viscera. A few others travel from more rostral brainstem sites with the glossopharyngeal nerve (⇒ parotid gland), the facial nerve (⇒ salivary and lacrimal glands) and the oculomotor nerve (⇒ pupillary sphincter and ciliary muscle).

7. Visceral afferent fibers to the brainstem travel through the solitary tract and end in the nucleus of the solitary tract.

Afferent fibers from the thoracic and abdominal viscera reach the brainstem with the vagus nerve. They travel within the brainstem in the solitary tract of the rostral medulla, and end in the surrounding nucleus of the solitary tract. A smaller number of glossopharyngeal afferents follow a similar course in the CNS.

Neurons in the nucleus of the solitary tract participate in various visceral reflexes (e.g., automatic adjustment of respiratory and cardiovascular parameters) and also convey information directly or indirectly to the hypothalamus.

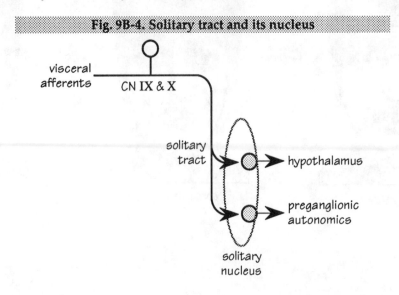

Fig. 9B-4. Solitary tract and its nucleus

8. Afferents from taste buds travel through the solitary tract and end in the nucleus of the solitary tract.

Afferents that innervate taste buds reach the brainstem with the facial nerve (from the anterior 2/3 of the tongue), the glossopharyngeal nerve (from the posterior 1/3 of the tongue) and the vagus nerve (from the epiglottis). They too travel within the brainstem in the solitary tract and end in the nucleus of the solitary tract, mostly in more rostral portions.

Gustatory neurons in the nucleus of the solitary tract participate in feeding and defensive activities like swallowing and coughing. They also convey information to the thalamus and thence to the cerebral cortex (conscious awareness of taste) and indirectly to the hypothalamus and amygdala (affective aspects of taste). Unlike most other ascending sensory pathways to the thalamus, the gustatory pathway is uncrossed.

Fig. 9B-5. Gustatory pathway

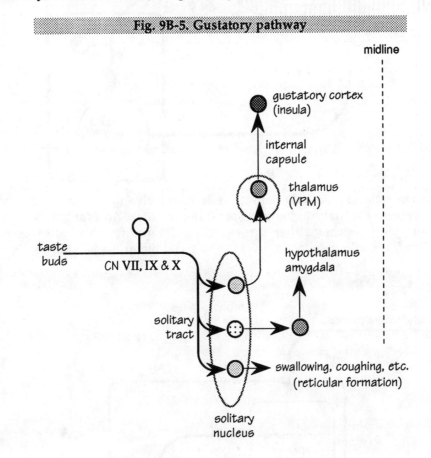

9. Cranial nerves are involved in stretch reflexes and withdrawal reflexes.

Cranial nerves are involved in a variety of reflexes, most of which are analogous to spinal cord reflexes. For example, stretching the masseter causes a reflex contraction by way of a monosynaptic circuit parallel to that of spinal stretch reflexes. The afferent cell bodies for this reflex are peculiar in that they reside within the CNS (in the mesencephalic trigeminal nucleus).

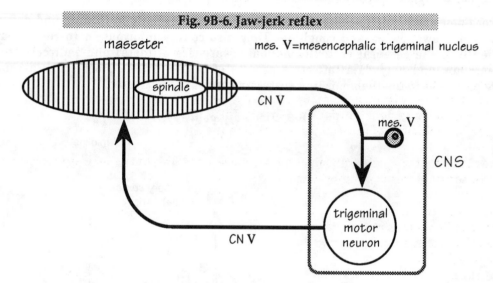

Fig. 9B-6. Jaw-jerk reflex

masseter

mes. V=mesencephalic trigeminal nucleus

Other brainstem reflexes, like other spinal reflexes, involve interneurons. Many of these reflexes are protective in nature, like the spinal flexor reflex. An example is blinking both eyes when an object touches either cornea. The afferents for this reflex travel in the trigeminal nerve, the efferents (cell bodies in the facial motor nucleus) in the facial nerve.

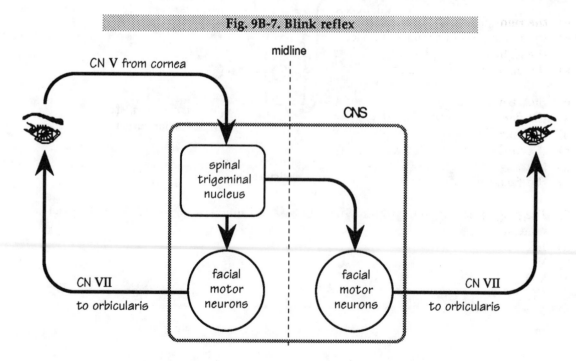

Fig. 9B-7. Blink reflex

1. The trigeminal nerve contains all of the following *except*
    a) motor axons to the masseter.
    b) primary afferents carrying gustatory information from taste buds in the back of the tongue.
    c) primary afferents carrying pain and temperature information from the forehead.
    d) primary afferents that end in the main sensory nucleus in the midpons.
    e) primary afferents from masseter muscle spindles.

2. Primary afferent fibers conveying pain and temperature information from the left side of the forehead terminate
    a) bilaterally in the spinal trigeminal nucleus.
    b) in the main sensory nucleus of the trigeminal nerve on the left side.
    c) in the spinal trigeminal nucleus of the left side.
    d) in the VPM nucleus of the thalamus on the right side.

3. Does the position of the trigeminal motor nucleus, relative to the main sensory nucleus, make sense in terms of embryology?

4. The most ventral part of the spinal trigeminal tract at the spinomedullary junction contains fibers that represent
    a) the middle of the forehead.
    b) the temple.
    c) the chin.
    d) the side of the jaw, near the ear.

5. Interruption of corticobulbar fibers in the left cerebral peduncle would result in weakness of
    a) the left side of the face.
    b) the right side of the face.
    c) the left lower quadrant of the face.
    d) the right lower quadrant of the face.
    e) the upper half of the face.

6. Motor neurons for the larynx and pharynx are located in
    a) the dorsal motor nucleus of the vagus.
    b) nucleus ambiguus.
    c) the nucleus of the solitary tract.
    d) the trigeminal motor nucleus.
    e) the facial motor nucleus.

7. Preganglionic parasympathetic fibers leave the brainstem in all of the following cranial nerves *except*
    a) III.
    b) V.
    c) VII.
    d) IX.
    e) X.

8. The nerve fibers of the solitary tract
  a) are central branches of facial, glossopharyngeal and hypoglossal fibers.
  b) convey gustatory and olfactory chemosensory information.
  c) mostly terminate in nucleus ambiguus.
  d) serve as the afferent limb of a variety of reflexes, including those that modulate cardiac and respiratory function.

9. Given that a patient had suffered damage to *either* one trigeminal nerve or one facial nerve, how could you determine which nerve was affected (and on which side), using one stroke of a wisp of cotton?

10. Trigeminal neuralgia is a condition of severe, intermittent pain in part of the trigeminal distribution. Total destruction of the trigeminal ganglion has been used as a treatment for this condition. What practical complications might arise from this treatment?

Answers and Explanations

1. **b**. These are in the glossopharyngeal nerve.

2. **c**. Primary afferents almost always end ipsilaterally, and do not reach the thalamus. The trigeminal main sensory nucleus subserves touch.

3. Yes, since the main sensory nucleus is dorsolateral to the motor nucleus, corresponding to their derivations from alar and basal plates.

4. **b**. See Fig. 9B-2.

5. **d**. See Fig. 9B-3.

6. **b**.

7. **b**. Contains somatic sensory fibers and motor axons to masseter and other muscles.

8. **d**. No hypoglossal fibers, no olfactory information; solitary tract terminates in the nucleus of the solitary tract.

9. Assuming only one of the four nerves is damaged, then when you stroke the left cornea:
   If both eyes blink, the left trigeminal and both facial nerves must be OK;
   if neither eye blinks, the left trigeminal nerve must be damaged;
   if only the left eye blinks, the right facial nerve must be damaged;
   if only the right eye blinks, the left facial nerve must be damaged.

10. Three examples: corneal abrasion from foreign objects due to loss of the blink reflex; chewing damage to the inside of the cheek, due to loss of sensation; drooling and loss of food from one side of the mouth, also due to loss of sensation. All these effects on the side ipsilateral to the treatment.

CHAPTER 9C

VESTIBULOCOCHLEAR NERVE

LEARNING OBJECTIVES

1. Differentiate between the bony and membranous labyrinths, and the fluids which fill various parts of them.

2. Describe or diagram the path taken by a sound wave from the outer to the inner ear. Indicate the roles of the tympanic membrane and the middle ear ossicles in transferring sound energy efficiently into the fluids of the inner ear.

3. Describe or diagram the mechanical arrangement of receptors and accessory structures in the cochlea which specialize it for responding to sound.

4. Diagram the central auditory pathway, indicating the sites of "obligatory" synapses and the locations where damage could cause unilateral deafness.

5. Describe the mechanical arrangement of receptors and accessory structures in the semicircular ducts and vestibule which determine the kinds of stimuli to which these parts of the labyrinth respond.

6. Name the principal routes through which the vestibular system can influence posture and eye movements. Indicate the origin and course of the vestibulospinal tracts.

7. Explain how optokinetic, rotatory, postrotatory and caloric nystagmus work, including an explanation of the direction of nystagmus in each case.

8. Explain the relevance of the retina and of neck proprioceptors to the integrated functioning of the vestibular system.

The eighth nerve is the nerve of hearing and equilibrium. All of its receptive functions are accomplished by variations on a common theme; the different sensory information carried by different fibers in the nerve is simply the result of slight differences in the mechanical arrangement of receptors and accessory structures.

1. The membranous labyrinth, filled with endolymph, is surrounded by perilymph and suspended within the bony labyrinth.

Eighth nerve fibers innervate special receptors called hair cells, located in an elaborate end organ called the labyrinth. The labyrinth is two series of twisted tubes (hence the name labyrinth), one suspended inside the other. The outer tube, the bony labyrinth, is a continuous channel in the temporal bone. The bony cochlea is located anteriorly, the bony semicircular canals posteriorly, and the vestibule between the two. The inner tube, the membranous labyrinth, is a second continuous tube suspended within the bony labyrinth; in the case of the cochlea, the mechanical arrangement of the suspension is crucial to the function of the end organ. The membranous labyrinth generally parallels portions of the bony labyrinth (i.e., there are cochlear and semicircular ducts), except that the vestibule contains two parts of the membranous labyrinth, the utricle and the saccule.

The bony labyrinth is filled with perilymph, which is more or less equivalent to cerebrospinal fluid. The membranous labyrinth, in contrast, is filled with endolymph, whose ionic composition more closely resembles that inside a cell (i.e., high $[K^+]$, low $[Na^+]$). The sensory hairs of the hair cells, the characteristic receptor cells of the labyrinth, poke through the wall of the membranous labyrinth and are typically inserted into a mass of gelatinous material. Relative movement of a hair bundle and the gelatinous material causes a depolarizing or a hyperpolarizing receptor potential (depending on whether the hair bundle is deflected toward or away from its tallest hair). This in turn causes an increase or a decrease in the release of an excitatory transmitter, and a consequent increase or decrease in the firing rate of any eighth nerve fiber that innervates the hair cell. The way in which the gelatinous material is arranged within the labyrinth plays a major role in determining the kind of mechanical stimulus to which a particular region of the labyrinth responds best.

Fig. 9C-1. Overview of labyrinth

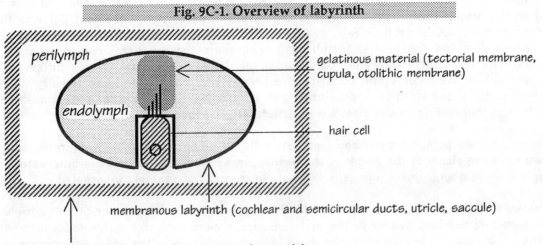

92

2. The tympanic membrane and middle ear ossicles effectively couple airborne sound vibrations to the fluid-filled inner ear.

Sound vibrations are funneled through the outer ear and vibrate the tympanic membrane. This in turn vibrates the malleus, incus and stapes (the middle ear ossicles), and the stapes footplate vibrates the perilymph of the inner ear through the oval window. (Inward pushes and outward pulls of the stapes are accommodated by outward and inward bulges of the round window membrane.) This elaborate mechanism is necessary because sound does not cross an air-water interface very well and there is essentially an air-water interface between the outside world and the perilymph of the cochlea. The slight mechanical advantage of the middle ear ossicles, together with the much larger area of the tympanic membrane relative to the oval window, results in a much greater force *per unit area* at the oval window than at the tympanic membrane.

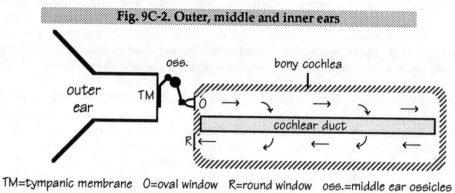

Fig. 9C-2. Outer, middle and inner ears

TM=tympanic membrane O=oval window R=round window oss.=middle ear ossicles

3. Vibratory deformation of the basilar membrane results in deflection of the sensory hairs of cochlear hair cells.

The cochlear duct is stretched as a partition across the cochlear part of the bony labyrinth. The partition is complete except for a small hole at the apex of the cochlea (the helicotrema) at which two subdivided perilymphatic spaces communicate with each other. Therefore when the stapes pushes inward part of the resulting perilymph movement deforms the cochlear duct. Cochlear hair cells are located in the organ of Corti in one wall of the cochlear duct (on the basilar membrane), with their sensory hairs embedded in the gelatinous tectorial membrane. Deformation of the cochlear duct causes differential movement of the basilar and tectorial membranes and this deflects the sensory hairs, which in turn causes either a depolarizing or a hyperpolarizing receptor potential in the hair cells (depending on the direction of deflection).

There are two populations of cochlear hair cells all along the basilar membrane. Inner hair cells are closer to the center of the cochlea, less numerous, but heavily innervated by eighth nerve fibers. Outer hair cells are more numerous but sparsely innervated.

Portions of the cochlear duct nearer to the oval window are more sensitive to higher frequencies; portions nearer to the helicotrema are more sensitive to lower frequencies. This is, at least to a great extent, the result of gradual changes in the width and mechanical properties of the basilar membrane.

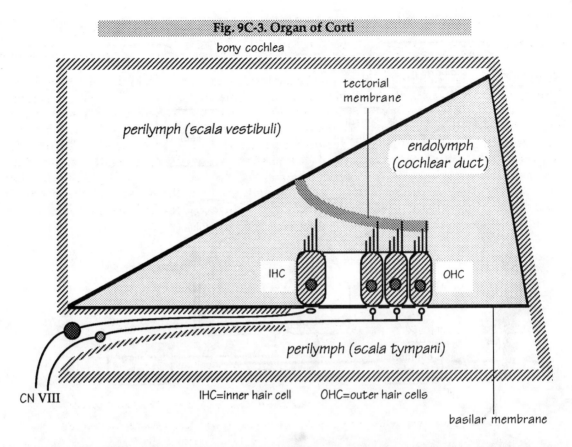

Fig. 9C-3. Organ of Corti

bony cochlea

tectorial membrane

perilymph (scala vestibuli)

endolymph (cochlear duct)

IHC

OHC

perilymph (scala tympani)

CN VIII

IHC=inner hair cell   OHC=outer hair cells

basilar membrane

4. Auditory information reaches the cochlear nuclei and from there is transferred bilaterally, in several stages, to auditory cortex.

We use our ears not only to identify sounds, but also to localize them in space. This localization is achieved by comparing the time and intensity differences in the sounds arriving at our two ears, and this comparison begins to be made early in the CNS. Cochlear nerve fibers end ipsilaterally, in the cochlear nuclei at the pontomedullary junction. The cochlear nuclei then project bilaterally in the brainstem, so that at all levels rostral to the cochlear nuclei each ear is represented bilaterally, and unilateral damage does not cause deafness of either ear. Rostral to the cochlear nuclei, the auditory pathway on each side is concerned not so much with one ear as with information from both ears relevant to the contralateral half of the auditory world.

Successively more rostral stages in the auditory pathway include the superior olivary nucleus (crossing fibers reach it through the trapezoid body), inferior colliculus (by way of the lateral lemniscus), medial geniculate nucleus of the thalamus (by way of the brachium of the inferior colliculus, or inferior brachium) and auditory cortex (part of the superior temporal gyrus).

94

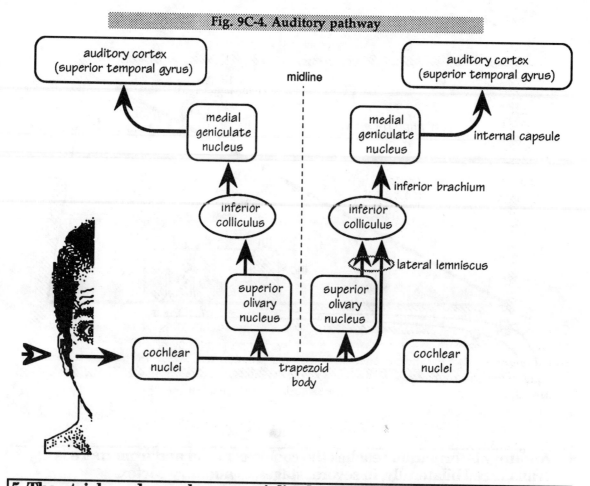

Fig. 9C-4. Auditory pathway

5. The utricle and saccule are specialized to respond to linear acceleration, whereas the semicircular ducts are specialized to respond to angular acceleration.

The utricle and saccule each contains a flattened patch of hair cells (a macula) overlain by a layer of gelatinous material containing crystals of calcium carbonate (hence called an otolithic membrane, or a "membrane full of ear stones"). The otolithic membrane is more dense than endolymph and so tries to move through it in response to gravity or other linear accelerations. This in turn deflects the hair bundles inserted into the otolithic membrane and elicits depolarizing or hyperpolarizing receptor potentials. The utricular macula is oriented in a mostly horizontal plane, the saccular macula in a mostly vertical plane. Hence the utricle is most sensitive to tilts beginning from a head-upright position, the saccule to tilts beginning from a head-sideways position.

The semicircular ducts use a different mechanism. Each contains a dilatation called an ampulla, in which the hair cells reside as part of a ridge called a crista. The hair bundles are inserted into a gelatinous diaphragm called a cupula. Movement of the endolymph within a semicircular duct would therefore distort the cupula and deflect the hair bundles.

95

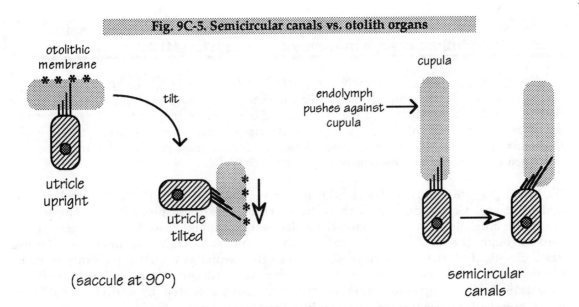

Fig. 9C-5. Semicircular canals vs. otolith organs

The most effective stimulus for causing such movement is angular acceleration in the plane of a given canal (like a wheel on an axle). For example, at the beginning of rotation the endolymph lags behind because of inertia and pushes on the cupula in one direction; at the end of rotation it continues to move, again because of inertia, and pushes on the cupula in the opposite direction.

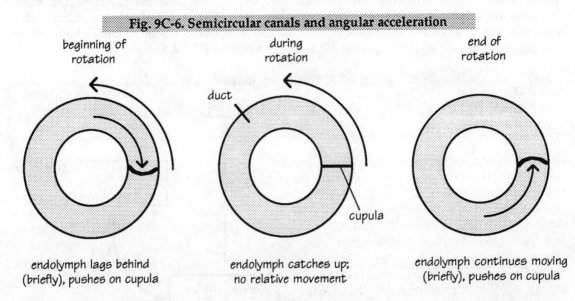

Fig. 9C-6. Semicircular canals and angular acceleration

There are three semicircular canals and ducts on each side, in three orthogonal planes. Roughly speaking, one is horizontal, one extends anteriorly at 45° to the sagittal plane, and one extends posteriorly at 45° to the sagittal plane. Hence rotation in any plane can be detected by each set of semicircular canals.

6. The vestibular system influences posture through the vestibulospinal tracts and influences eye movements through the MLF.

Vestibular primary afferents mostly end in the vestibular nuclei although some reach the cerebellum directly (the only primary afferents that get to the cerebellum; primarily to the flocculonodular lobe). Outputs from the vestibular nuclei go mostly to places that make sense from a functional point of view. There is a vestibular projection through the thalamus to the cerebral cortex (parietal lobe), but for the most part vestibular projections influence posture and eye movements.

We make postural adjustments in response to vestibular stimuli like tilts, accelerations and rotations. Corresponding to this, there are two vestibulospinal tracts. The medial vestibular nucleus projects a bilateral medial vestibulospinal tract to the cervical spinal cord through the MLF. The lateral vestibular nucleus sends the uncrossed lateral vestibulospinal tract to all cord levels. We use the medial vestibulospinal tract to make compensatory neck movements, and the lateral vestibulospinal tract to make postural adjustments in antigravity muscles. Both are supplemented by indirect vestibular nuclei➔reticular formation➔reticulospinal tract projections.

We can keep our eyes pointed at something even if we're moving around. That is, a head movement of 30° to the left can be automatically nulled by a conjugate eye movement of 30° to the right. For slow head movements with your eyes open this is partly a visual tracking movement, but you can do it even in the dark, and you can do it while your head is moving faster than visual tracking movements can work. The additional basis for these compensatory eye movements is the vestibuloocular reflex, a simple three-neuron reflex arc. Vestibular primary afferents project to the vestibular nuclei, which then project (mostly, but not entirely, through the MLF) to the nuclei of III, IV and VI.

Fig. 9C-7. Vestibular connections

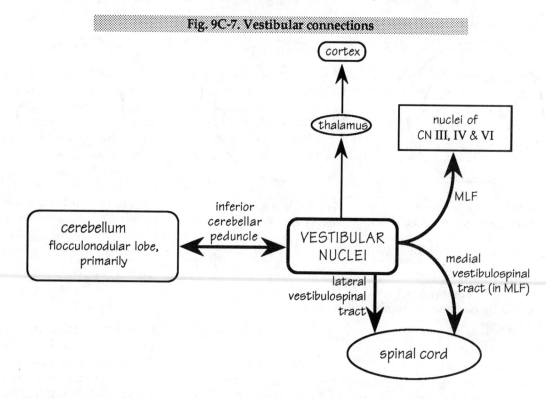

7. Reflex attempts to maintain visual stability can result in nystagmus.

Consider in a little more detail what would happen at the beginning of rotation to your left in the dark. At first, the vestibuloocular reflex would move your eyes to the right, the appropriate movement to keep the direction in which your eyes are pointed from changing (i.e., to keep your gaze from shifting). However, there is obviously a limit to how far your eyes can rotate in their sockets, and if you continue to spin around then these compensatory movements are periodically interrupted by fast "reset" movements in the opposite direction. The combined back-and-forth movement is called nystagmus, and it gets named for the direction of the fast component. Hence at the beginning of rotation to the left there would be nystagmus to the left ("left-beating nystagmus"). If rotation is maintained in the dark, the vestibular stimulus loses its effectiveness (Fig. 9C-6) and the rotatory nystagmus ceases. Right after a rotation terminates, the direction of cupula deflection is the opposite of that at the beginning of rotation (Fig. 9C-6), and so there is postrotatory nystagmus in the opposite direction.

The same nystagmus can be elicited by moving a repetitive visual stimulus in front of someone. In this case it is called optokinetic nystagmus. The nystagmus at the beginning of rotation with the lights on is a combination of rotatory and optokinetic nystagmus (both in the same direction, since both are reflex attempts to maintain visual stability). If the rotation continues with the lights on, optokinetic nystagmus may persist.

Stimulating one horizontal semicircular canal is sufficient to cause nystagmus, and this can be done calorically using warm or cool water. With the head tilted back so that the horizontal canal is in an approximately vertical plane, cool water in one ear causes nystagmus with its fast phase to the opposite side and warm water causes nystagmus with its fast phase to the same side (text Fig. 9-40, p. 221).

8. The vestibular, visual and somatosensory systems function together to provide a unified perception of orientation and movement.

The vestibular system plays a major role, but not the only role, in our ability to sense and maintain our orientation with respect to gravity, as well as in our ability to maintain visual fixation while we move. Contrary to what you might think, the thing it's most indispensable for is helping with eye movements. People with bilateral vestibular loss recover to a point where their sense of orientation is pretty good, but they continue to have trouble maintaining gaze unless they move relatively slowly.

We actually use three different sensory systems to tell us about position and movement—vestibular, visual and somatosensory (especially neck receptors). People can do pretty well with only two of these systems, and that's the basis for compensation after loss of vestibular function. If two of the three systems aren't working, we have a lot of trouble. For example, someone with no vestibular function or deficient somatosensory function would be very disabled in the dark. The three systems can interact in sometimes surprising ways: visual-vestibular conflicts can cause striking illusions of movement; neck dysfunction can cause nystagmus.

Information from these three systems needs to be integrated at an early stage. As one example, the semicircular canals can only signal maintained rotation for a little while, but the postural adjustments need to be maintained or you fall down. As a second example, if you were resting your head on your desk and your chair started to slide out, you'd probably make postural adjustments even though there had been no vestibular input. This integration starts to happen at the level of the vestibular nuclei, which up until now we have pretended received only vestibular and cerebellar inputs. In fact, the same cells receive somatosensory and visual inputs. In the first example, visual inputs to the vestibular nuclei cause continued nystagmus (called optokinetic nystagmus in this case, since it is maintained by moving visual stimuli) and postural adjustments just as the original vestibular signal did. In the second example, the neck-vestibular mismatch would cause a vestibulospinal output.

Self-Evaluation Questions

1. The membranous labyrinth
a) is filled with perilymph.
b) includes the vestibule.
c) includes the saccule.
d) (a) and (c).
e) none of the above.

2. Hair cells that synapse on eighth nerve fibers
a) have sensory hairs bathed in endolymph.
b) can produce both hyperpolarizing and depolarizing receptor potentials, depending on the direction in which their hair bundles are deflected.
c) all work by having fluid currents deflect their hair bundles.
d) (a) and (b).
e) all of the above.

3. The most important factor in efficient transfer of sound energy into the inner ear is
a) the relative sizes of the tympanic membrane and the oval window.
b) the mechanical advantage provided by the middle ear ossicles.
c) funneling of sound by the outer ear.
d) the ionic composition of perilymph, which allows sound to cross an air-perilymph interface with great efficiency.

4. Endolymph
a) fills the utricle.
b) bathes the synapses between hair cells and eighth nerve fibers.
c) has a sodium concentration similar to that of cerebrospinal fluid.
d) flows through the helicotrema.

5. Outer hair cells
a) are found exclusively near the apex of the cochlea, accounting for the fact that the apex of the cochlea is most sensitive to high frequencies.
b) are found exclusively near the apex of the cochlea, accounting for the fact that the apex of the cochlea is most sensitive to low frequencies.
c) are found at all levels of the cochlea; the increased sensitivity of the apex of the cochlea to high frequencies is caused by other factors.
d) are found at all levels of the cochlea; the increased sensitivity of the apex of the cochlea to low frequencies is caused by other factors.

6. The gelatinous substance into which cochlear hair bundles are inserted is called the
a) tectorial membrane.
b) otolithic membrane.
c) cupula.
d) basilar membrane.

7. Both ears are represented in all of the following nuclei *except* the
a) superior olivary nucleus.
b) inferior colliculus.
c) cochlear nuclei.
d) medial geniculate nucleus.
e) Both ears are represented in all of these nuclei.

8. Primary auditory cortex is located in
a) the parietal lobe, just posterior to the postcentral gyrus.
b) the lateral surface of the occipital lobe.
c) the superior temporal gyrus.
d) the inferior temporal gyrus.
e) the middle frontal gyrus.

9. Holding your head tilted forward 15° would most effectively stimulate hair cells in the
a) utricle.
b) saccule.
c) semicircular ducts.

10. Interactions among the vestibular, visual and somatosensory systems first occur in the
a) parietal lobe.
b) vestibular nuclei.
c) spinal cord.
d) occipital lobe.
e) temporal lobe.

11. A mad neuroanatomist built an apparatus for demonstrating the activity of the vestibular system, and somehow persuaded a local fish trainer to try it out. The fish trainer crawled into a horizontal tube, laid down on his back, and rested his head on a 30° wedge so that his head was tilted upward. The neuroanatomist turned out the lights and turned on a motor that spun the tube on its long axis, to the fish trainer's right, and then left the room for a while. Electrical recordings of the fish trainer's eye movements showed
a) nystagmus to the left (fast phase) for several seconds, then a period of no nystagmus, then nystagmus to the right when the rotation stopped.
b) nystagmus to the left for the duration of the rotation, then nystagmus to the right when the rotation stopped.
c) nystagmus to the right for several seconds, then a period of no nystagmus, then nystagmus to the left when the rotation stopped.
d) nystagmus to the right for the duration of the rotation, then nystagmus to the left when the rotation stopped.
e) nystagmus to the left throughout the rotation, and for several seconds after the rotation stopped.

100

Answers and Explanations

1. **c.** Perilymph *surrounds* the membranous labyrinth; the vestibule is part of the bony labyrinth, and contains the saccule and utricle.

2. **d.** See Fig. 9C-1.

3. **a.** The mechanical advantage of the ossicles is slight.

4. **a.** Endolymph has a high $[K^+]$ and low $[Na^+]$, and synapses could not work in this environment. The helicotrema connects two perilymph-filled compartments.

5. **d.** The basilar membrane is broader and looser toward the apex of the cochlea, and so resonates at lower frequencies.

6. **a.** See Fig. 9C-3 (or text Fig. 9-34, p. 213).

7. **c.** Cochlear primary afferents end uncrossed in the cochlear nuclei. At all levels rostral to this, information from both ears is compared.

8. **c.**

9. **a.** The semicircular ducts respond best to changes in angular velocity, the saccule to tilts starting from a head-sideways position.

10. **b.** See Section 8 in this chapter.

11. **c.** Vestibular nystagmus does not persist during maintained rotation. See Fig. 9C-6 (or text Fig. 9-40, p. 221).

CHAPTER 10

DIENCEPHALON

LEARNING OBJECTIVES

1. Describe or diagram the general pattern of connections between the cerebral cortex, the thalamus, and other subcortical sites.

2. Describe the topographic division of the thalamus into major nuclear groups.

3. Compare and contrast the specific relay nuclei and the association nuclei of the thalamus. List the specific relay nuclei and, for each, indicate its major input and the cortical area to which it projects. Identify the large expanses of association cortex in the human brain, and indicate the thalamic nucleus with which each is connected.

4. Name the major forebrain structures between which the internal capsule is located. Indicate how these structures are used as landmarks to divide the internal capsule into portions, and list the principal contents of each of these portions.

5. Describe the general relationships between the hypothalamus and the anterior and posterior lobes of the pituitary gland.

The major components of the diencephalon, the thalamus and hypothalamus, are active in practically everything we do. The thalamus is the gateway to the cerebral cortex, and the hypothalamus regulates autonomic function and drive-related behavior.

1. The thalamus is the major source of afferents to the cerebral cortex.

Some collections of chemically coded fibers, such as serotoninergic fibers and noradrenergic fibers from the brainstem, reach the cerebral cortex directly. However, the vast majority of the afferents to the cerebral cortex arise in the thalamus (or in the cortex itself). These thalamocortical afferents include fibers representing all the specific sensory, motor and limbic pathways. In contrast, efferents from the cerebral cortex to sites like the spinal cord, brainstem and basal ganglia reach their targets directly. (Although there are also many cortical efferents back to the thalamus, these do not form part of any descending pathway.) This large collection of cortical afferents and efferents travels through the internal capsule.

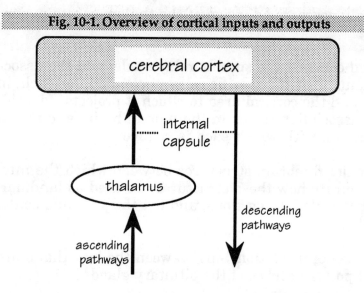

Fig. 10-1. Overview of cortical inputs and outputs

2. The thalamus is divided into lateral, medial and anterior nuclear groups.

A thin sheet of myelinated fibers, the internal medullary lamina, subdivides the thalamus into nuclear groups. The internal medullary lamina bifurcates anteriorly and so defines anterior, medial and lateral nuclear groups. In addition, the lateral and medial geniculate nuclei (LGN and MGN) form two bumps posteriorly and inferiorly on the main bulk of the thalamus.

The anterior and medial subdivisions each has only one major nucleus (the anterior and dorsomedial nuclei, respectively). The lateral division, in contrast, contains an array of four major nuclei or nuclear groups. From anterior to posterior these are the ventral anterior nucleus (VA), the ventral lateral nucleus (VL), the ventral posterolateral and ventral posteromedial nuclei (VPL/VPM), and the pulvinar.

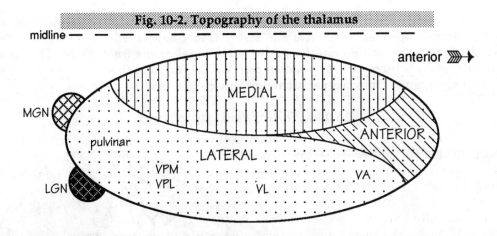

Fig. 10-2. Topography of the thalamus

3. The thalamus contains some nuclei that project to specific functional areas of the cerebral cortex and others that project to association areas.

The thalamic nuclei that form part of specific functional systems receive particular bundles of afferents and project heavily to particular cortical areas with more or less well-defined functions. These nuclei are therefore referred to as specific relay nuclei. The major examples of specific relay nuclei, with their inputs and outputs, are indicated in Fig. 10-3.

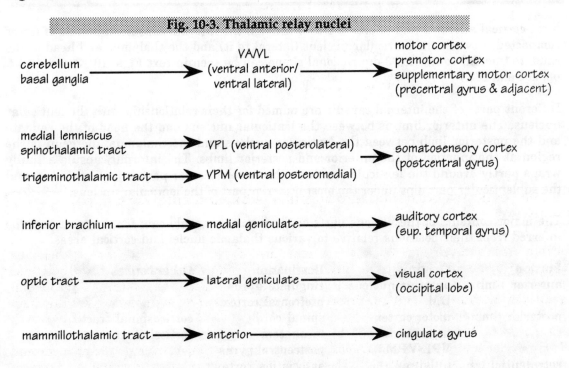

Fig. 10-3. Thalamic relay nuclei

104

Most of the cortical areas not accounted for in the projections of the specific relay nuclei form two large expanses of association cortex (see Chapter 15). The first, prefrontal association cortex, is located anterior to the motor areas of the frontal lobe. The second is the parietal-occipital-temporal association cortex. Each of these fields of association cortex receives major inputs from its own thalamic association nucleus.

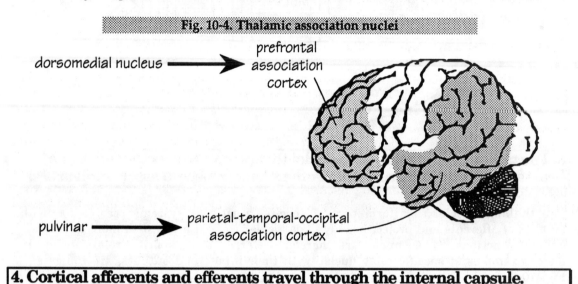

Fig. 10-4. Thalamic association nuclei

dorsomedial nucleus ⟶ prefrontal association cortex

pulvinar ⟶ parietal-temporal-occipital association cortex

4. Cortical afferents and efferents travel through the internal capsule.

Most cortical afferents and efferents travel through the internal capsule, a bundle of fibers compacted between the lenticular nucleus (lateral to it) and the thalamus and head of the caudate (medial to it). (Its 3-dimensional shape can be seen in text Figs. 10-13 and 10-14, pp. 262 and 263.)

Different parts of the internal capsule are named for their relationship with the lenticular nucleus. The anterior limb is between the lenticular nucleus and the head of the caudate and the posterior limb between the lenticular nucleus and the thalamus; the genu is the region at the junction of the anterior and posterior limbs. The internal capsule actually wraps partly around the lenticular nucleus; the retrolenticular part is just behind it, and the sublenticular part dips under the most posterior part of the lenticular nucleus.

The major contents of the various parts of the internal capsule can, for the most part, be inferred from their positions relative to various thalamic nuclei and cortical areas.

Portion	Origin	Destination	Other Names
anterior limb	anterior nucleus	cingulate gyrus	
	DM	prefrontal cortex	
posterior limb	motor cortex	spinal cord	corticospinal tract
	motor cortex	brainstem	corticobulbar tract
	VPL/VPM	postcentral gyrus	
retrolenticular	pulvinar	association cortex	
	LGN	visual cortex	optic radiation
sublenticular	LGN	visual cortex	optic radiation
	MGN	auditory cortex	auditory radiation

5. The hypothalamus controls the output of the pituitary gland through both neurosecretory and humoral routes.

Parts of the hypothalamus are exposed at the base of the brain, surrounded by the circle of Willis. The mammillary bodies form the most posterior part of the hypothalamus, and lie adjacent to the cerebral peduncles. Between the mammillary bodies and the optic chiasm and tract is the tuber cinereum. The median eminence arises from the tuber cinereum and narrows into the infundibular stalk, to which the pituitary gland is attached.

The hypothalamus is a major control center for the autonomic nervous system. It therefore has extensive interconnections with visceral sensory and motor nuclei, as well as with various limbic structures (see Chapter 16), especially the hippocampus, amygdala and septal area. In addition, the hypothalamus controls the pituitary gland (hypophysis) through two separate mechanisms. 1) Hypothalamic neurons in the supraoptic and paraventricular nuclei are the source of antidiuretic hormone (vasopressin) and oxytocin. They transport these hormones down their axons to the posterior lobe of the pituitary (neurohypophysis), where they are released into the circulation. 2) Hypothalamic neurons in the tuber cinereum produce small peptides that serve as releasing and inhibiting factors for the anterior pituitary (adenohypophysis). They transport these factors down their axons and release them into capillaries in the median eminence. These capillaries then converge into pituitary portal vessels which travel down the infundibular stalk to a second capillary bed in the anterior pituitary. The releasing and inhibiting factors leave the second capillary bed and control the production of anterior pituitary hormones.

Fig. 10-5. Hypothalamic control of the pituitary gland

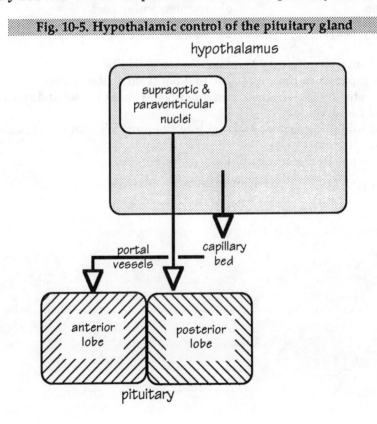

Self-Evaluation Questions

For questions 1–7, match the connections in the column on the left with the thalamic nuclei in the column on the right; a given thalamic nucleus may be used more than once or not at all.

1. inputs from medial lemniscus
2. outputs to prefrontal cortex
3. outputs to occipital lobe
4. outputs to postcentral gyrus
5. inputs from mammillothalamic tract
6. outputs to superior temporal gyrus
7. outputs to precentral gyrus

a) anterior nucleus
b) VL
c) medial geniculate nucleus
d) dorsomedial nucleus
e) VPL
f) lateral geniculate nucleus

For questions 8–11, match the fiber types in the column on the left with the parts of the internal capsule in the column on the right; for each fiber type, use as many parts as apply.

8. efferents from anterior nucleus
9. corticospinal tract
10. optic radiation
11. somatosensory fibers

a) anterior limb
b) posterior limb
c) retrolenticular part
d) sublenticular part

12. Production of anterior pituitary hormones is controlled by
a) direct neural input from the supraoptic and paraventricular nuclei.
b) hormones secreted by the supraoptic and paraventricular nuclei and released into hypothalamic blood vessels.
c) releasing and inhibiting factors secreted into the pituitary portal circulation by hypothalamic neurons.
d) direct neural input from neurons in the tuber cinereum.

Answers and Explanations

1. **e.** Somatosensory relay nucleus for the body.

2. **d.** Association nucleus for prefrontal cortex.

3. **f.** Relay nucleus for vision.

4. **e.** Somatosensory relay nucleus for the body.

5. **a.** Limbic relay nucleus.

6. **c.** Auditory relay nucleus.

7. **b.** Motor relay nucleus.

8. **a.** On their way to the cingulate gyrus.

9. **b.**

10. **c, d.**

11. **b.** Posterior limb is adjacent to VPL.

12. **c.** See Fig. 10-5 (or text Fig. 10-19, p. 255).

CHAPTER 11

VISUAL SYSTEM

LEARNING OBJECTIVES

1. Diagram schematically the major cell types of the retina and their synaptic relationships.

2. Describe the distinguishing anatomical features of the fovea and the optic disk, and indicate the functional correlates of these features.

3. Diagram the pathway leading from the retina to visual cortex, and describe the retinotopic map in visual cortex.

4. Given a drawing of someone's visual fields, indicate whether the fields are normal or abnormal. If abnormal, name the deficit and indicate which part of the nervous system might have been damaged to produce the deficit.

5. Diagram the neural pathways controlling pupillary size, and indicate where in these pathways damage might cause a dilated pupil or a constricted pupil.

6. Diagram the neural circuits involved in the pupillary light reflex and the near (accommodation) reflex.

The visual system is the most studied sensory system, partly because we are such a visually oriented species and partly because of its *relative* simplicity. In addition, the visual pathway is highly organized in a topographical sense, so that even though it stretches from the front of your face to the back of your head, damage anyplace causes deficits that are relatively easy to understand.

1. The retina contains five major cell types arranged in orderly layers.

The job of the retina is to convert patterns of light into trains of action potentials in the optic nerve. It does this using five basic cell types, whose cell bodies are arranged in three layers (outer and inner nuclear layers, ganglion cell layer). Alternating with these three layers of cell bodies are an outer and an inner plexiform layer where the synaptic interactions occur. In the outer plexiform layer photoreceptor cells (rods and cones) bring visual information in, bipolar cells take it out, and horizontal cells mediate lateral interactions. In the inner plexiform layer bipolar cells bring visual information in, ganglion cells take it out (their axons form the optic nerve), and amacrine cells mediate lateral interactions.

Fig. 11-1. Retinal organization

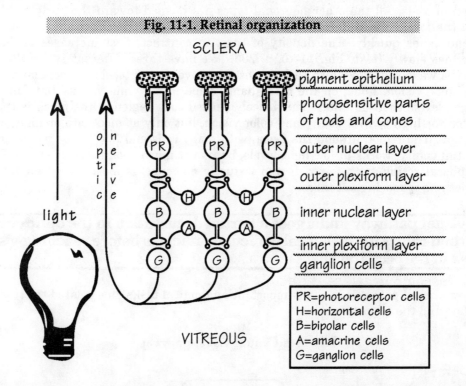

Standard descriptions of the retina as a ten-layered structure also include a row of junctions between adjacent photoreceptors (outer limiting membrane), the layer of ganglion cell axons (nerve fiber layer), and the basal lamina on the vitreal surface of the retina (inner limiting membrane). Notice that the last part of the retina reached by light is the photosensitive parts of the rod and cone cells, embedded in processes of pigment epithelial cells.

2. The retina contains a fovea specialized for color vision and high acuity, and a blind spot where optic nerve fibers leave the eye.

Ganglion cell axons travel along the vitreal surface of the retina, and so they need to pierce the sclera to leave the eye in the optic nerve. They do so by converging on the optic disk, slightly medial to the optic axis, turning 90° posteriorly, and leaving the eye. Here the optic nerve acquires a dural sheath continuous with the dural covering of the CNS. (The dural sheath is lined with arachnoid and contains a bit of subarachnoid space; increases in intracranial pressure are therefore transmitted along the optic nerve and cause papilledema, or swelling of the optic disk.) Since there are no photoreceptors at the optic disk, it corresponds to a blind spot in the visual field of each eye. The optics of the eye reverse images on the retina, so the blind spot of each eye lies on the horizontal meridian of the visual field, slightly *lateral* to the midline.

The center of the visual field corresponds to the fovea, a small retinal region in the middle of a pigmented zone called the macula. The fovea is packed with thin, densely packed cones and no rods. All the other neuronal types are pushed toward the periphery, so the center of the fovea is a small pit (text Fig. 11-8, p. 283). Outside the fovea, the number of cones diminishes quickly. The density of rods, in contrast, first increases rapidly and then declines slowly (text, Fig. 11-10, p. 285). We have three different types of cones in terms of the wavelength to which each is most sensitive, so the total cone population can be used for color vision. Rods, on the other hand, come in only one variety but function at lower light levels than do cones. The densely packed cone region of the fovea is therefore specialized for high spatial acuity and color vision, but only at moderate or high levels of illumination. The region around the fovea, with many rods and few cones, has reasonably good spatial acuity, works at low light levels, but is not much good for color vision. Finally, the peripheral retina, with few rods and virtually no cones, is mostly good for telling us that something is moving out there.

3. The visual pathway undergoes a partial decussation in the optic chiasm, and then relays in the lateral geniculate nucleus before reaching visual cortex in the occipital lobe.

The central visual pathway has two important anatomical tasks, one related to crossings of the midline and the other to maps.

Fig. 11-2. Central visual pathway

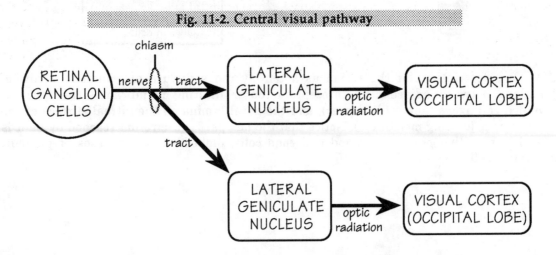

Since our eyes face forward their visual fields overlap to a great extent (text Fig. 11-21, p.302), so it would make sense for information from *each retina* about the contralateral half of the visual world to reach a given side of the brain. This is accomplished by a partial decussation of the optic nerves in the optic chiasm, in which the ganglion cell axons from the nasal half of each retina cross the midline and join undecussated fibers from the temporal half of the contralateral retina in the optic tract. (For example, since the optics of the eye reverse things, the temporal half of the left retina and the nasal half of the the right retina both "look at" the right half of the visual world.) This separation of the visual world into two halves is maintained in the rest of the visual pathway. The optic tract ends in the lateral geniculate nucleus of the thalamus. The lateral geniculate gives rise to the optic radiation, which passes through the retrolenticular and sublenticular parts of the internal capsule and ends in primary visual cortex above and below the calcarine sulcus.

As in the case of other sensory systems, the visual system maintains an orderly map of the information it carries and emphasizes in this map certain functionally important regions. In this case, the visual pathway maintains a retinotopic map of the image falling on each retina, with a disproportionately large number of fibers representing the fovea. The mapping culminates in primary visual cortex, where the *retina* is represented right side up (i.e., superior *fields* below the calcarine sulcus, inferior fields above), the fovea posteriorly at the occipital pole and the periphery anteriorly. The foveal representation, relative to the size of the fovea, is much larger than the representation of the periphery.

4. Damage to various parts of the visual pathway causes predictable deficits.

Knowledge of the visual pathway enables one to predict the deficits resulting from damage anyplace in the pathway; knowledge of a little terminology allows one to name them (Fig. 11-3). Deficits are generally named for the visual field affected. Heteronymous means the affected fields of the two eyes do not overlap, and homonymous means the affected fields overlap to a greater or lesser degree. Therefore, damage in front of the optic chiasm affects only the eye ipsilateral to the damage, damage to the optic chiasm generally causes heteronymous deficits, and damage behind the chiasm causes homonymous deficits. Terms like hemianopia and quadrantanopia mean half or a quarter of a visual field is nonfunctional.

Fibers on their way to the upper bank of the calcarine sulcus go through the retrolenticular part of the internal capsule and straight back to the occipital lobe. Fibers on their way to the lower bank go through the sublenticular part and loop out into the temporal lobe (Meyer's loop) before turning posteriorly toward the occipital lobe (text Fig. 11-14A, p. 289). Damage in the optic radiation or the occipital lobe sometimes spares part of the large foveal representation, resulting in foveal or macular sparing.

112

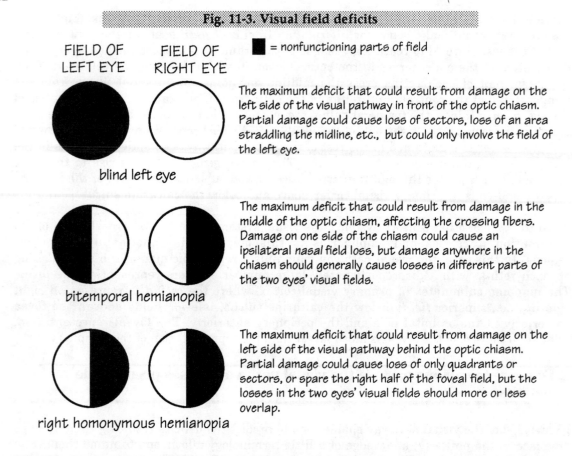

Fig. 11-3. Visual field deficits

FIELD OF LEFT EYE   FIELD OF RIGHT EYE   ■ = nonfunctioning parts of field

blind left eye

The maximum deficit that could result from damage on the left side of the visual pathway in front of the optic chiasm. Partial damage could cause loss of sectors, loss of an area straddling the midline, etc., but could only involve the field of the left eye.

bitemporal hemianopia

The maximum deficit that could result from damage in the middle of the optic chiasm, affecting the crossing fibers. Damage on one side of the chiasm could cause an ipsilateral *nasal* field loss, but damage anywhere in the chiasm should generally cause losses in different parts of the two eyes' visual fields.

right homonymous hemianopia

The maximum deficit that could result from damage on the left side of the visual pathway behind the optic chiasm. Partial damage could cause loss of only quadrants or sectors, or spare the right half of the foveal field, but the losses in the two eyes' visual fields should more or less overlap.

5. The iris receives both sympathetic and parasympathetic innervation.

The size of the pupil is determined by the balance between a relatively strong sphincter and a relatively weak dilator (Fig. 11-4). The sphincter receives parasympathetic innervation via the oculomotor nerve and the ciliary ganglion, and is normally activated during the pupillary light reflex and the near reflex (next section). The dilator receives sympathetic innervation via the intermediolateral cell column of the spinal cord and the superior cervical ganglion. The preganglionic sympathetic neurons for the dilator can be activated by long descending pathways from the ipsilateral half of the hypothalamus, as well as by other routes.

Pupils of significantly unequal size usually signify damage to some aspect of the autonomic innervation of one eye or to the iris itself. A dilated pupil (mydriasis), unresponsive to all stimuli, could be caused by damage to the ipsilateral oculomotor nerve. Such damage, if it affected the entire nerve, would also be accompanied by weakness of the other muscles supplied by the third nerve, most prominently ptosis (because of a weak levator palpebrae) and lateral strabismus (because of an unopposed lateral rectus). A pupil that was relatively constricted (=miosis), but still responsive to light shone through it, could be caused by damage to either its preganglionic or its postganglionic sympathetic innervation, or to fibers on the ipsilateral side of the brainstem as they descend from the hypothalamus to the spinal cord. (In the pons and medulla, the latter fibers are located near the spinothalamic tract.) This would constitute part of Horner's syndrome, and would be accompanied by slight ipsilateral ptosis (weakness of the sympathetically innervated tarsal muscles) but not by any weakness of extraocular muscles.

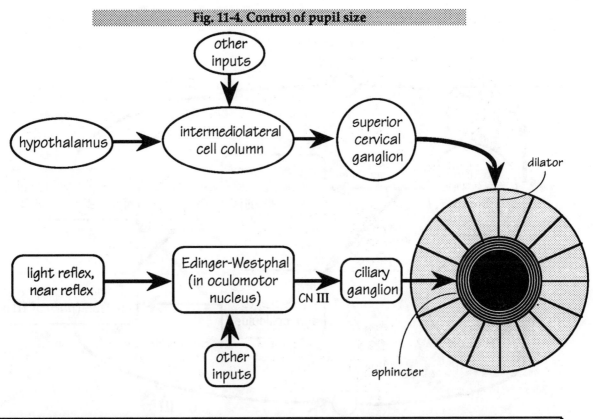

Fig. 11-4. Control of pupil size

---

6. Increased illumination and near objects both elicit visual reflexes.

A commonly tested cranial nerve reflex is the pupillary light reflex (Fig. 11-5). Light shone through one pupil causes both sphincters to contract equally. The response of the illuminated eye is the direct reflex, the equal response of the unilluminated eye the consensual reflex. Afferent impulses for this reflex arc travel over ganglion cell axons in the optic nerve; half of them cross in the optic chiasm. However, they bypass the lateral geniculate nucleus and travel instead through the superior brachium to the pretectal area, just rostral to the superior colliculus at the midbrain-diencephalon junction. Fibers from the pretectal area then distribute bilaterally to the Edinger-Westphal subnucleus of the oculomotor nucleus, where the preganglionic parasympathetic neurons live. Because of the bilateral distribution of fibers both in the optic chiasm and in going from pretectal area to oculomotor nucleus, light in one eye causes equal constriction of both pupils. Optic nerve damage produces equal pupils, neither one of which responds to light shone into the eye ipsilateral to the damage, but both of which respond normally to light shone into the contralateral eye. Oculomotor nerve damage, in contrast, causes a dilated ipsilateral pupil that does not respond to light shone into either eye.

114

Fig. 11-5. Pupillary light reflex

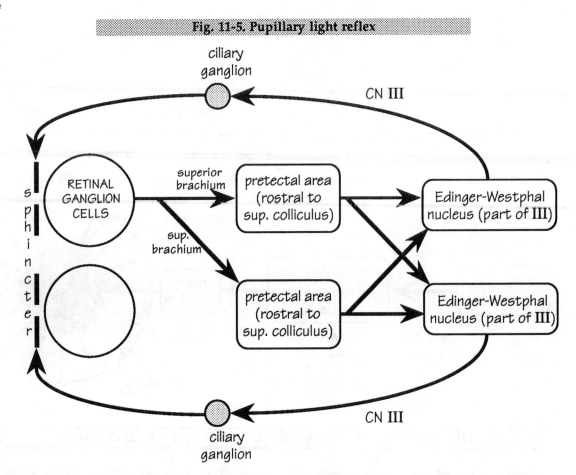

Looking at something nearby causes three things to happen in reflex fashion: 1) both medial recti contract, converging the eyes; 2) both ciliary muscles contract, allowing the lens to fatten and thus focus the image of the nearby object on the two retinas; 3) both pupillary sphincters contract, improving the optical performance of the eye. Since this near reflex or accommodation reflex typically involves consciously looking at something, it is not surprising that its pathway involves a loop through visual cortex (Fig. 11-6). The afferent limb is the standard visual pathway through the lateral geniculate nucleus and visual cortex. After one or more synapses in the occipital lobe, the efferent limb involves a projection back through the superior brachium to the pretectal area and/or the superior colliculus and from there to the oculomotor nucleus. (The stop in the superior colliculus is omitted from Fig. 11-6 for simplicity.)

115

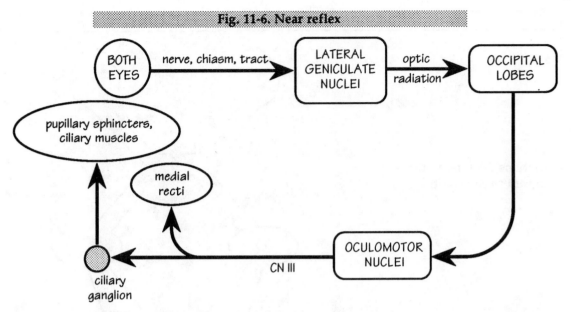

Fig. 11-6. Near reflex

Questions 1-5 refer to the diagram to the right.

Match the visual field defects shown to the right with the letters of the lesions shown above, using each letter only once.

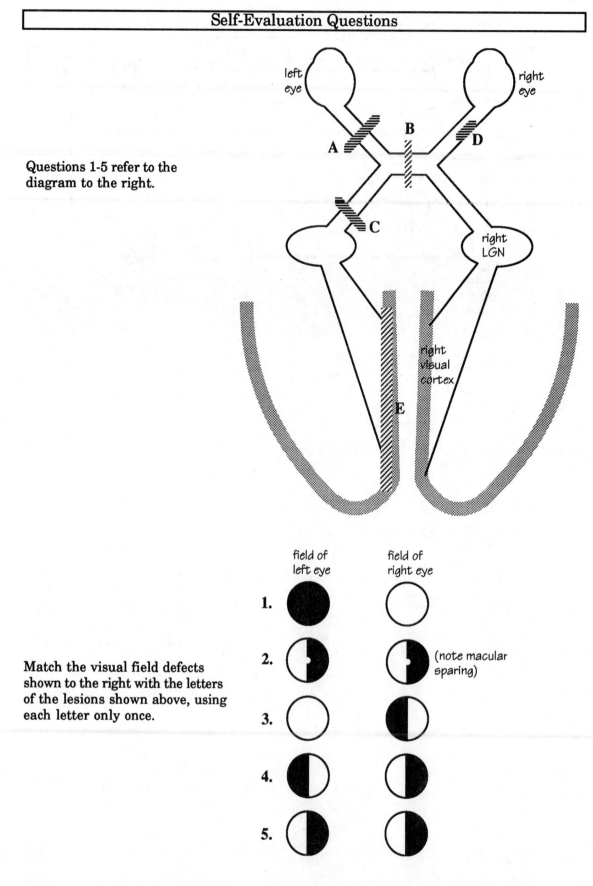

6. Lateral interactions in the inner plexiform layer are mediated by
a) horizontal cells.
b) amacrine cells.
c) bipolar cells.
d) ganglion cells.

7. Relative to the representation of the fovea in the visual field, the blind spot is
a) medial.
b) lateral.
c) superior.
d) inferior.

8. Our color vision is best for images that fall on
a) the fovea.
b) the region of the retina surrounding the fovea.
c) the peripheral retina.

9. Right superior homonymous quadrantanopia could be caused by damage to
a) the sublenticular part of the right internal capsule.
b) the retrolenticular part of the right internal capsule.
c) the sublenticular part of the left internal capsule.
d) the retrolenticular part of the left internal capsule.

10. The representation of the left half of each fovea is located
a) posteriorly in the right occipital lobe.
b) posteriorly in the left occipital lobe.
c) anteriorly on the medial surface of the right occipital lobe.
d) anteriorly on the medial surface of the left occipital lobe.

11. A large pupil that does not respond to light shone in either eye could be the result of damage to the
a) contralateral lateral horn of the spinal cord.
b) ipsilateral oculomotor nerve.
c) ipsilateral optic nerve.
d) either (b) or (c).
e) any of the above.

12. A person who suffers from congenital absence of retinal rods would have little difficulty in seeing the picture on a color television, but would have great difficulty in seeing the picture on a black-and-white television.
a) True.
b) False.

13. Bilateral damage to the occipital lobes would abolish
a) the pupillary light reflex.
b) the near reflex.
c) both reflexes.
d) neither reflex.

118

Answers and Explanations

1. **a.** Left optic nerve damage→blind left eye.

2. **e.** Left visual cortex damage→right homonymous hemianopia, often with macular sparing.

3. **d.** Right nasal hemianopia: only one eye affected, so it must be due to a lesion in front of the optic chiasm or on the side of the optic chiasm.

4. **b.** Damage to crossing fibers in the optic chiasm (from nasal halves of the retinas)→bitemporal hemianopia.

5. **c.** Left optic tract damage→right homonymous hemianopia.

6. **b.** See Fig. 11-1.

7. **b.** The optic nerve leaves the back of the eye a little medial to the fovea. Since the optics reverse everything, the blind spot is a little lateral to the fovea in the visual field. See text Fig. 11-21, p. 302.

8. **a.** The fovea is a region of tightly packed cones.

9. **c.** Fibers on their way to the lower bank of the calcarine sulcus, representing upper quadrants of the visual field, pass through the sublenticular part of the internal capsule.

10. **b.** See text Fig. 11-15, pp. 292 and 293.

11. **b.** Asymmetrical pupils usually mean damage to the motor nerves supplying the iris. A large pupil implies an unopposed dilator, caused by oculomotor damage; lack of a light response confirms this. (Another possibility is damage to the iris itself.)

12. **b.** Cones are not *forced* to subserve color vision. For example, you are using your foveas to read this black and white book.

13. **b.** See Figs. 11-5 and 11-6.

CHAPTER 12

CORTICOSPINAL AND CORTICOBULBAR TRACTS

LEARNING OBJECTIVES

1. List the principal descending pathways that influence the activity of spinal cord motor neurons.

2. Describe the locations of the cortical areas that give rise to the corticospinal tract, and indicate the orientation of the homunculus in primary motor cortex.

3. Define spasticity, list any clinical signs that commonly accompany spasticity, and indicate the parts of the CNS whose damage causes this condition. Compare and contrast the effects of upper motor neuron disease and lower motor neuron disease.

4. Describe the corticobulbar innervation of cranial nerve nuclei, paying particular attention to the patterns of bilateral or predominantly crossed projections from motor cortex to these nuclei.

5. Compare and contrast saccadic, tracking and vergence eye movements. Indicate which cortical areas are involved in each.

The firing rates of our motor neurons, and therefore the states of contraction of our muscles, are determined by multiple influences. Simple reflex arcs like the stretch reflex and more complex "motor programs" like the basic pattern generator for walking are built into the spinal cord and brainstem. These reflex arcs and motor programs, as well as the motor neurons themselves, are in turn influenced by various descending pathways. Finally, activity in the descending pathways is modulated by the basal ganglia (Chapter 13) and the cerebellum (Chapter 14).

1. Descending tracts from the cerebral cortex, vestibular nuclei, reticular formation and red nucleus influence spinal cord motor neurons.

The principal pathway mediating voluntary movement is the corticospinal tract, a direct projection from cerebral cortex to spinal cord (together with an analogous corticobulbar tract from cerebral cortex to cranial nerve motor nuclei). Corticospinal fibers originate from several adjacent cortical areas (see next section), descend through the internal capsule, cerebral peduncle, basal part of the pons, and the medullary pyramid of each side. Most of these fibers then cross the midline in the pyramidal decussation to form the lateral corticospinal tract (the few uncrossed fibers form the anterior corticospinal tract).

Destruction of the corticospinal tract does not cause total paralysis, so there must be other descending pathways through which movements can be initiated. The major alternative is a collection of reticulospinal fibers from the brainstem reticular formation to the spinal cord. In addition, vestibulospinal tracts mediate postural adjustments and the small rubrospinal tract assists in the control of distal muscles. The rubrospinal tract, like the corticospinal tract, crosses the midline before terminating. Reticulospinal projections are bilateral, and vestibulospinal projections are primarily uncrossed.

Fig. 12-1. Major descending pathways

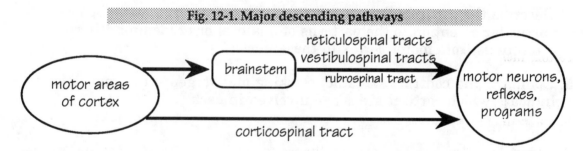

2. Motor, premotor, supplementary motor and somatosensory cortex are somatotopically arranged and project fibers through the corticospinal tract.

Corticospinal fibers originate from cortical areas near the central sulcus. Many arise in motor cortex in the precentral gyrus and in premotor cortex, just anterior to the precentral gyrus. Both areas are arranged somatotopically, so that neurons projecting to cranial nerve motor neurons are most ventral, those projecting to leg motor neurons are near the top of the central sulcus, and those projecting to arm and hand motor neurons are in between. Particularly large areas are devoted to the hand and mouth. In addition, some corticospinal fibers arise in the supplementary motor area on the medial surface of the hemisphere and others arise in the postcentral gyrus (somatosensory cortex).

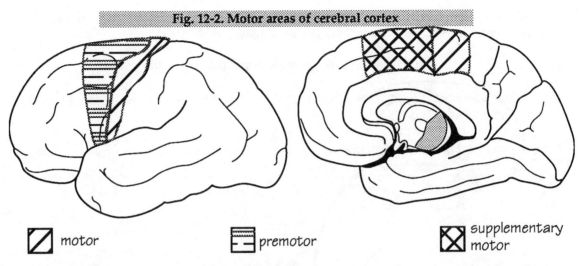

Fig. 12-2. Motor areas of cerebral cortex

⬜ motor   ⬜ premotor   ⬜ supplementary motor

3. Corticospinal damage typically results in weakness, increased tone and hyperactive stretch reflexes.

Corticospinal (and corticobulbar) neurons, also called upper motor neurons, can be damaged in cortical lesions. The result is spastic hemiparesis, in which the contralateral side of the body is weak, stretch reflexes are increased, and muscle tone is increased. The flexors of the upper extremity and the extensors of the lower extremity are particularly affected. Babinski's sign (dorsiflexion of the big toe in response to stroking the sole of the foot) is also present on the side contralateral to the lesion, and clonus (rhythmic contractions in response to maintained muscle stretch) may also be seen. The increased tone collapses abruptly in response to strong efforts to overcome it (clasp-knife response).

Spastic hemiparesis is the result of massive disruption of the output from motor areas of the cortex, including outputs to the brainstem reticular formation. Hence it can result from damage to the cerebral cortex, the posterior limb of the internal capsule, or the spinal cord (where corticospinal and other descending fibers are intermingled to some extent). On the other hand, damage only to primary motor cortex or selective damage to the corticospinal fibers in the pyramid causes weakness and Babinski's sign, but not spasticity.

Spasticity is markedly different from the results of lower motor neuron damage, i.e., damage to the motor neurons themselves. Lower motor neuron disease is also accompanied by weakness, but in this case reflexes and tone are diminished. In addition, the weak muscles fasciculate and atrophy.

4. Cranial nerve motor nuclei typically receive bilateral corticobulbar innervation, but there are important exceptions.

Fibers of the upper motor neurons for cranial nerve motor nuclei form the corticobulbar tract (Fig. 12-3). These fibers mostly accompany the corticospinal tract until they reach the level of the nuclei in which they terminate. In contrast to corticospinal fibers, however, they are distributed bilaterally to a great extent. The result is that, with one major exception, corticobulbar damage on one side does not cause contralateral weakness of muscles innervated by cranial nerves. The major exception is the muscles of the lower face, whose motor neurons are innervated predominantly by contralateral cerebral cortex, with the result that corticobulbar damage on one side causes contralateral weakness of only the lower face. In addition, the trigeminal and hypoglossal nuclei receive more

122

crossed than uncrossed fibers in many individuals, and corticobulbar damage can result in slight contralateral weakness of the jaw or tongue.

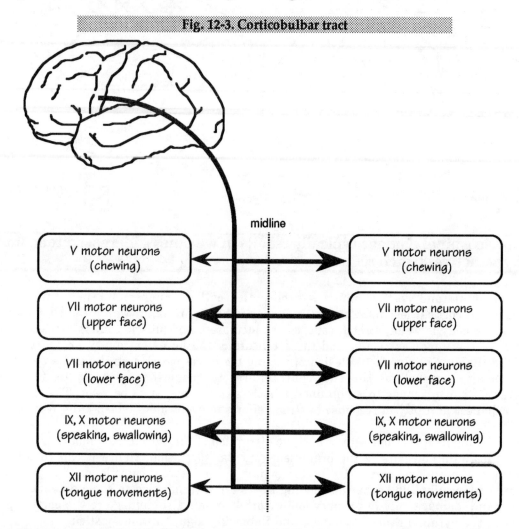

Fig. 12-3. Corticobulbar tract

5. Different cortical areas are involved in fast and slow conjugate eye movements and in vergence movements.

We automatically try to keep our eyes pointed in such a way that each bit of the image of the outside world falls on corresponding points on our two retinas. This accomplishes two things: it gets the image of whatever we're interested in onto the fovea for best acuity, and allows for depth perception. If the system breaks down and the two images don't correspond, diplopia (double vision) results.

Two general kinds of movements are required to keep our eyes lined up this way while we move or the world moves. First, as things move around at a given distance from us we need to move both eyes the same amount in the same direction; these are called conjugate movements. Second, as things move toward us or away from us we need to either converge or diverge our eyes; these are appropriately called vergence movements. In addition, we make two different kinds of conjugate movements: slow movements, which we use to track slowly moving objects, and fast movements called saccades, which we use when something moves too fast to track or when there is nothing to track.

It would be nice if all we needed to do for eye movements was send a bunch of timing signals from someplace like motor cortex to the motor neurons in the oculomotor, trochlear and abducens nuclei. However, it's a little more complicated than that. We have groups of subcortical neurons specialized to generate the timing signals—basically, the motor programs for eye movements. These timing centers receive inputs from those parts of the brain that can "order" eye movements, and then send their outputs to the motor neurons. Superimposed on this arrangement are projections from the vestibular nuclei, so that we can adjust eye position to compensate for head movements.

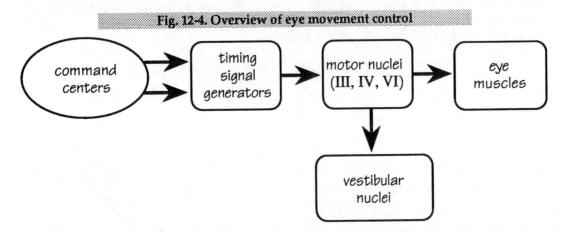

Fig. 12-4. Overview of eye movement control

Conjugate movements. The arrangement for vertical conjugate movements is reasonably straightforward. The superior and inferior recti, both innervated by the oculomotor nerve, are the principal muscles. (For the sake of simplicity, the trochlear nerve and its nucleus are omitted from this account). Corresponding to this, the motor neurons and most of the timing machinery live in the midbrain. The cells that devise the timing signals for upward movements are located near the superior colliculi and posterior commissure and are distributed bilaterally. (Things that press on the top of the midbrain, like pineal tumors, commonly cause a selective paralysis of upward gaze.) The timing signals for downward gaze come from deeper in the midbrain, near the dorsomedial edge of the red nucleus. Here again, bilateral lesions are required for function to be disrupted.

For horizontal conjugate movements, things aren't quite that simple, because we need to coordinate the lateral rectus of one eye with the medial rectus of the other eye. This is accomplished by having not only motor neurons in each abducens nucleus, but also interneurons that project through the MLF to the oculomotor nucleus (Chapter 9A). The vestibular nuclei also project via the MLF to the oculomotor, trochlear and abducens nuclei so that we can maintain gaze while moving our heads around (this is the vestibuloocular reflex).

Saccades are rapid conjugate movements, in which our eyes can move as rapidly as 700°/second. We use saccades for voluntary eye movements, or to look over at something we caught a glimpse of in the periphery, or to catch up with something that's moving too fast to track. Moving your eyes like this is harder than it seems. It requires a very rapid burst (up to 1000 impulses/second) in the motor neurons to generate the velocity, and then requires a carefully calculated maintained firing rate to keep the eyes in their new position. For vertical saccades, these timing signals are generated in the midbrain as described earlier. For horizontal saccades, the timing signals are generated in the paramedian pontine reticular formation (PPRF). The PPRF on one side of the pons sets up the signals for saccades to the ipsilateral side. Saccades are prepackaged movements, as though the brain calculates how far we need to move, sets up the timing, and then lets it fly.

Once it starts, the saccade usually can't be changed, if for example the target moves again. One of the few ways a saccade can be modified is through the vestibular nuclei. If you move your head during a saccade, the vestibuloocular reflex automatically compensates for the movement.

We use pursuit or tracking movements to track a moving object once its image is on or near the fovea. Pursuit movements can go at a maximum rate of only 50°/second or so. As a result, rapidly or irregularly moving objects require a combination of saccades and pursuit movements. Also, there's a latency of about 125 msec for pursuit movements when a target starts to move, so by the time we start to track something, its image has moved off the fovea; in such cases a catchup saccade is required.

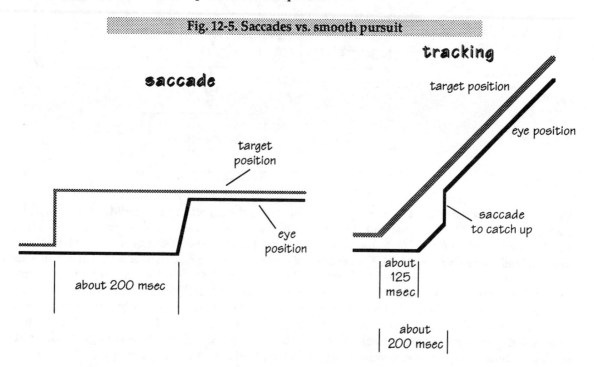

Fig. 12-5. Saccades vs. smooth pursuit

Since saccades are used primarily in voluntary eye movements, it is not surprising that they are triggered from the frontal lobes. There is a specific area, called the frontal eye field, just anterior to where the head is represented in motor cortex. Vertical eye movements are apparently represented bilaterally, since a unilateral frontal lesion causes no problems with vertical saccades. In the case of horizontal saccades, each hemisphere triggers movements to the contralateral side. However, after unilateral frontal lesions, even horizontal saccades recover quickly (usually in a matter of days). How much of this recovery depends on the other frontal lobe, and how much depends on the superior colliculus, is unclear.

We know much less about the neural machinery for pursuit movements than we do for saccades. They're usually said to be triggered from visual association cortex in the occipital lobes, but posterior parts of the temporal lobe seem more likely. As in the case of saccades, vertical movements are triggered bilaterally. Oddly enough, one hemisphere seems to trigger horizontal pursuit movements primarily to the *ipsilateral* side. The pathway from cortex to the abducens and oculomotor nuclei may involve stops in the flocculus and the vestibular nuclei, since damage at both these sites disrupts pursuit movements.

Vergence movements. Vergence movements are part of the near reflex, described in Chapter 11. The afferent limb of the reflex is the normal visual pathway from eyeball to occipital lobe. Visual association cortex of the occipital lobe then projects to the efferent machinery in the midbrain.

Fig. 12-6. Cortical control of eye movements

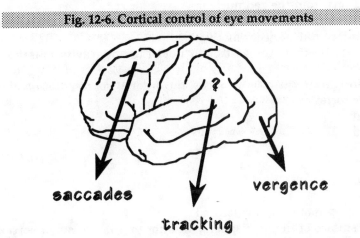

1. Descending influences on spinal cord motor neurons include all of the following *except*
   a) crossed projections from the red nucleus.
   b) crossed projections from the ventral lateral (VL) nucleus of the thalamus.
   c) bilateral reticulospinal projections.
   d) uncrossed projections from the vestibular nuclei to antigravity muscles.

2. Moving superiorly from the lateral sulcus, the order of representation of body parts in primary motor cortex is
   a) leg, arm, head.
   b) arm, leg, head.
   c) arm, head, leg.
   d) leg, head, arm.
   e) head, arm, leg.

3. The supplementary motor area is located
   a) on the medial surface of the hemisphere, anterior to primary motor cortex.
   b) on the medial surface of the hemisphere, posterior to primary motor cortex.
   c) on the lateral surface of the hemisphere, anterior to primary motor cortex.
   d) in the parietal lobe, posterior to somatosensory cortex.
   e) on the lateral surface of the hemisphere, anterior to premotor cortex.

4. Upper motor neuron disease and lower motor neuron disease are similar in that in both conditions
   a) stretch reflexes are diminished.
   b) muscles fasciculate and atrophy.
   c) the flexors of the upper extremity are affected more than the extensors.
   d) Babinski's sign is present.
   e) none of the above.

5. Spasticity on the right would be likely after damage to the
   a) left frontal lobe.
   b) posterior limb of the left internal capsule.
   c) left lateral funiculus of the spinal cord.
   d) either (a) or (b).
   e) all of the above.

6. The pathway and apparatus for the near reflex include all of the following *except* the
   a) oculomotor nucleus.
   b) visual cortex.
   c) MLF.
   d) pupillary sphincter.
   e) ciliary muscle.

7. Damage to motor cortex on one side typically causes some contralateral weakness when
   a) speaking.
   b) swallowing.
   c) raising eyebrows.
   d) smiling.

8. A 39-year-old handball hustler comes to you complaining of the sudden onset of
    difficulty reading the sports pages, because he can't make his eyes move from left to
    right. You confirm that he cannot seem to look to his right on command, but notice that
    his eyes can move to the right when you roll a handball across the floor. The most
    likely site of damage is his
a) left frontal lobe.
b) right frontal lobe.
c) left abducens nucleus.
d) right abducens nucleus
e) could be either (a) or (d).

Answers and Explanations

1. **b**. The thalamus only projects to other forebrain structures, particularly the cerebral
    cortex.

2. **e**. See text Fig. 12-3, p. 308.

3. **a**. See Fig. 12-2.

4. **e**. **a** and **b** are characteristics of lower motor neuron disease, **c** and **d** of upper motor
    neuron disease.

5. **d**. Corticospinal fibers cross in the pyramidal decussation.

6. **c**. Convergence does not require medial rectus-lateral rectus coordination.

7. **d**. Motor neurons for muscles of the larynx, pharynx and upper face receive bilateral
    corticobulbar innervation.

8. **a**. Voluntary eye movements (saccades) to the contralateral side are triggered from the
    frontal eye field. Tracking movements involve more posterior cortical areas. Damage
    to the abducens nucleus would affect both types of movement. (Another possible site of
    damage to account for this problem would be the right PPRF.)

CHAPTER 13

BASAL GANGLIA

LEARNING OBJECTIVES

1. List the basal ganglia. Indicate the terms used for different combinations of the basal ganglia, and the combining forms of these various terms that are used to name pathways involving the basal ganglia.

2. Describe the conformation and location of the caudate nucleus, putamen, globus pallidus, subthalamic nucleus and substantia nigra.

3. Diagram the major circuit through which the basal ganglia affect the cerebral cortex. Name and describe the fiber bundles through which the globus pallidus projects to the thalamus.

4. Compare and contrast, in a general sense, the connections of the caudate nucleus and the putamen.

5. Diagram or describe the major connections of the substantia nigra and the subthalamic nucleus with the remaining basal ganglia.

6. Distinguish among chorea, athetosis, tremor and ballism. Indicate which of these are associated with damage at specific anatomical sites.

7. Describe the kinds of lesions that cause spasticity and rigidity, and differentiate between these two conditions.

Historically, the basal ganglia have been considered as major components of the motor system. In fact, they have a much broader role than that and are probably involved to some extent in most or all forebrain functions. However, their relationship to movement is their best understood aspect, and that is what shows up clinically in disorders like Parkinson's disease and Huntington's chorea. The interrelationships of the basal ganglia and motor areas of the cerebral cortex are emphasized in this chapter, but you should keep in mind that the basal ganglia have extensive connections, similar in principle and parallel in detail, with most other areas of the cerebral cortex.

1. The major basal ganglia are the caudate nucleus, putamen, globus pallidus, substantia nigra and subthalamic nucleus.

The meaning of the term "basal ganglia" has changed over the years, but most folks would now agree that there are five major structures on the list: caudate nucleus, putamen, globus pallidus, substantia nigra and subthalamic nucleus. The caudate and putamen have similar but parallel connections and are referred to in combination as the striatum. The putamen and globus pallidus have very different connections but are physically stuck together; in combination, they are referred to as the lenticular nucleus (from the Latin word for lentil). Finally and unfortunately, because of its appearance in stained sections, the combination of caudate and lenticular nuclei is sometimes referred to as the *corpus striatum*.

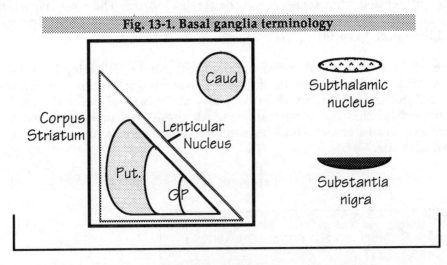

Fig. 13-1. Basal ganglia terminology

BASAL GANGLIA

The terms "strio-" and "-striate" are used to refer to fibers coming from or going to the striatum; for example, corticostriate fibers start in the cerebral cortex and end in the caudate or putamen. Similarly, the terms "pallido-" and "-pallidal", "nigro-" and "-nigral", and "subthalamo-" and "-subthalamic" are used to refer to fibers coming from or going to the globus pallidus, the substantia nigra or the subthalamic nucleus.

2. The basal ganglia are located in the telencephalon, diencephalon and midbrain.

The caudate nucleus parallels the lateral ventricle, having an enlarged head in the wall of the anterior horn, a smaller body adjacent to the body of the ventricle, and a still smaller tail adjacent to the inferior horn.

The lenticular nucleus (putamen+globus pallidus) underlies the insula and is shaped like a wedge cut from a sphere (text Figs. 13-1 and 13-2, pp. 320–321). The globus pallidus is the more medial, tapering part of the wedge, extending toward the interventricular foramen and thalamus. The caudate and putamen merge with each other anteriorly at the base of the septum pellucidum (text Fig. 16-5B, p. 398); the area of fusion is the nucleus accumbens (see text Chapter 16).

The substantia nigra is mostly located in the rostral midbrain, between the basis pedunculi (of the cerebral peduncle) and the red nucleus; part of it extends rostrally just into the diencephalon.

The subthalamic nucleus, as its name implies, is located inferior to the thalamus, just above the most rostral part of the substantia nigra.

3. The caudate and putamen receive cortical inputs and in turn influence the cortex by way of the globus pallidus and thalamus.

How does damage to the basal ganglia cause movement (and other) disorders? For the most part, we know only the broad outlines of an answer, but there is one basic fact to keep in mind: *the basal ganglia have no major outputs to lower motor neurons.* Instead, they work primarily by influencing what comes out of the cerebral cortex. The most important set of anatomical connections through which this happens is a loop from cortex through basal ganglia and then back to cortex.

The striatum is, in a sense, the input part of the basal ganglia, collecting information from large cortical areas (different areas for different parts of the striatum). The striatum then projects to the globus pallidus, which in turn projects by way of the thalamus back to a restricted portion of this large cortical area. All these structures, and most of their interconnections, are in one cerebral hemisphere, so damage to one of them results in contralateral deficits.

Fig. 13-2. Principal circuit of the basal ganglia

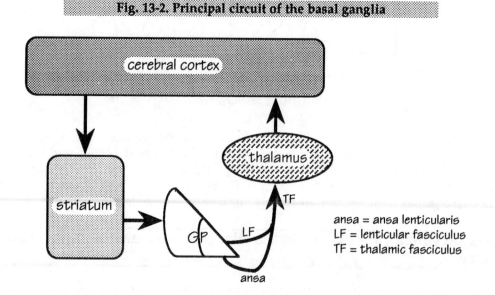

ansa = ansa lenticularis
LF = lenticular fasciculus
TF = thalamic fasciculus

Pallidal output fibers reach the thalamus through two bundles. The ansa lenticularis (text Figs. 13-11 and 13-13, pp. 328 and 330) hooks around the medial edge of the internal capsule. The lenticular fasciculus (text Fig. 13-12, p.329) passes directly through the internal capsule. The two bundles join cerebellar output fibers beneath the thalamus and form the thalamic fasciculus (text Figs. 13-11 and 13-12, pp. 328 and 329), which then enters the thalamus.

4. The putamen is primarily interconnected with sensorimotor cortex, the caudate nucleus with association cortex.

Although the cortex➤striatum➤globus pallidus➤thalamus➤cortex pathway is commonly drawn as a single loop, it is actually a system of parallel, overlapping loops, each wired up according to the same principles. Thus, the caudate nucleus receives its inputs from a different widespread area of the cortex than does the putamen, projects to its own part of the globus pallidus and from there to its own part of the thalamus and its own restricted cortical area.

The putamen subsystem is the part most directly involved in movement disorders. Its inputs come from the motor and somatosensory areas flanking the central sulcus. Its outputs reach the supplementary motor area by way of the ventral lateral and ventral anterior nuclei of the thalamus (VL and VA). This set of connections is consistent with the notion that the putamen and supplementary motor area are somehow involved in planning voluntary movements.

Fig. 13-3. Putamen connections

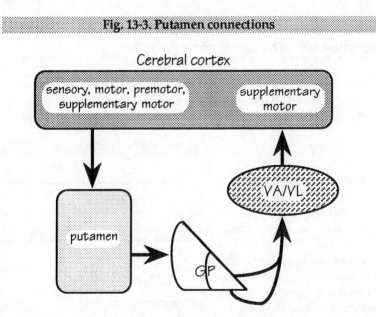

The caudate nucleus, in contrast, seems to be more involved in cognitive functions, although much less is known about how this involvement shows up in our day-to-day activities. Caudate inputs come from widespread association areas of the cerebral cortex and caudate outputs, by way of VA and the dorsomedial nucleus (DM), reach prefrontal cortex (Fig. 13-4). So the anatomical connections are appropriate for an involvement of the caudate in cognitive functions.

132

Fig. 13-4. Caudate connections

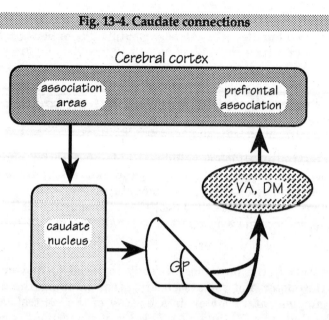

There's even a basal ganglia loop that involves the limbic system (described in Chapter 16 of the text).

5. The substantia nigra is interconnected with the striatum, the subthalamic nucleus with the globus pallidus.

The substantia nigra and the subthalamic nucleus do not participate directly in the cortex-striatum-cortex loop. Instead, each has reciprocal connections with other basal ganglia and each provides part of the substrate for an indirect route through the basal ganglia.

Fig. 13-5. Substantia nigra connections

The substantia nigra is connected primarily with the striatum. The pigmented neurons of the compact part of the substantia nigra (SNc) send dopaminergic fibers (DA) to the striatum. The reticular part of the substantia nigra (SNr) acts like a displaced part of the globus pallidus, receiving inputs from the striatum and projecting to the thalamus.

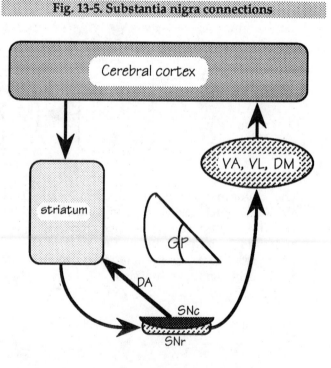

Fig. 13-6. Subthalamic nucleus connections

The subthalamic nucleus receives its major inputs from the external segment of the globus pallidus, and then projects to the internal segment of the globus pallidus. This provides an alternative route through the basal ganglia, as indicated in Fig. 13-6. The fibers that travel back and forth between the subthalamic nucleus and the globus pallidus penetrate the internal capsule as small bundles that are collectively called the subthalamic fasciculus (text Fig. 13-10, p. 327).

6. Basal ganglia lesions can cause movement disorders.

The best-known basal ganglia disorders are characterized by a combination of positive and negative signs—positive signs being involuntary muscle contractions in various patterns and negative signs being a lack of muscle contraction. Parkinson's disease is the classic example. Positive signs include a resting tremor, especially pronounced in the hands, and a general increase in tone in all muscles, referred to as rigidity. Negative signs include slow movements (bradykinesia) and few movements (hypokinesia or akinesia). There's no particular change in strength or reflexes. Other basal ganglia disorders can be accompanied by different kinds of involuntary movements that fall into three general categories: rapid movements called chorea, slow, writhing movements called athetosis, and flailing movements of an entire limb, called ballism. In some disorders, tone is increased even more than in Parkinson's; in others, it is decreased.

Disruption of the dopaminergic projection from the substantia nigra to the striatum is the cause of Parkinson's disease. Disruption of the connections between the globus pallidus and the subthalamic nucleus causes ballism on the contralateral side (i.e., contralateral hemiballismus).

7. The rigidity of Parkinson's disease and the spasticity of upper motor neuron disease are characterized by different symptoms and signs.

	Rigidity	Spasticity
Strength	unchanged	decreased
Reflexes	unchanged	increased
Tone	increased	increased
Distribution	all muscles	upper extremity flexors, lower extremity extensors
Other	resting tremor; hypokinesia; bradykinesia; cogwheeling	Babinski sign; clonus; clasp-knife response

Self-Evaluation Questions

1. The basal ganglia include all of the following *except* the
a) globus pallidus.
b) putamen.
c) substantia nigra.
d) thalamus.
e) subthalamic nucleus.

2. The term "strionigral fibers" could be used to refer to fibers that project from the
a) caudate nucleus to the substantia nigra.
b) substantia nigra to the putamen.
c) subthalamic nucleus to the substantia nigra.
d) globus pallidus to the substantia nigra.

3. The major source of inputs to the caudate nucleus is
a) the globus pallidus.
b) the subthalamic nucleus.
c) the putamen.
d) association areas of the cortex, like prefrontal cortex.
e) motor and somatosensory cortex.

4. The major circuit through which the basal ganglia affect the cerebral cortex involves a projection from
a) the globus pallidus to the thalamus.
b) the globus pallidus to the substantia nigra.
c) the striatum to the thalamus.
d) the striatum to the cerebral cortex.
e) the globus pallidus to the cerebral cortex.

5. Spasticity and parkinsonian rigidity are similar in that in both conditions there is
a) weakness.
b) increased stretch reflexes.
c) increased biceps tone.
d) tremor at rest.
e) none of the above.

6. A 39-year-old handball hustler noticed the abrupt onset of involuntary movements of his right side. His right arm and leg would make large, violent flailing movements that interfered with his game. The most likely site of damage was his
a) left substantia nigra.
b) right substantia nigra.
c) left globus pallidus.
d) right globus pallidus.
e) left subthalamic nucleus.
f) right subthalamic nucleus.

Answer questions 7–10 using the following diagram:

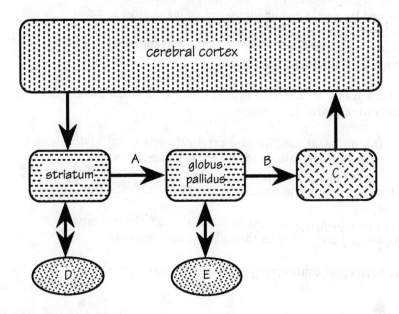

7. Lenticular fasciculus.

8. Thalamus.

9. Subthalamic nucleus.

10. Substantia nigra.

136

Answers and Explanations

1. **d.** See Fig. 13-1.

2. **a.** "Strio-" indicates that the fibers originate in the caudate or putamen; "-nigral" indicates that they end in the substantia nigra.

3. **d.** The caudate nucleus receives most of its cortical inputs from association areas, the putamen from somatosensory and motor areas.

4. **a.** See Fig. 13-2.

5. **c.** Rigidity is not characterized by weakness or increased reflexes, and spasticity is not characterized by tremor at rest. However, rigidity includes increased tone of most or all muscles and spasticity includes increased tone in upper extremity flexors. Thus, both conditions have increased biceps tone in common.

6. **e.** Flailing movements of both limbs on one side typifies hemiballismus. Basal ganglia disorders are seen contralateral to a lesion.

7. **b.** In the principal circuit linking basal ganglia and cerebral cortex, pallidothalamic fibers travel through the lenticular fasciculus and the ansa lenticularis.

8. **c.** The path from corpus striatum to cerebral cortex must pass through the thalamus.

9. **e.** Other than inputs from the striatum and outputs to the thalamus, the principal interconnections of the globus pallidus are with the subthalamic nucleus.

10. **d.** The striatum has major reciprocal connections with the substantia nigra.

CHAPTER 14

CEREBELLUM

LEARNING OBJECTIVES

1. Diagram the relationships of mossy fibers, granule cells, climbing fibers and Purkinje cells as the major input-output structures of the cerebellar cortex. Indicate the relationship between the cerebellar cortex and the deep cerebellar nuclei.

2. Describe or diagram the division of the cerebellum transversely into anterior, posterior and flocculonodular lobes, and longitudinally into hemispheral, intermediate and vermal zones. Indicate the connections of each of these longitudinal zones with the dentate, interposed and fastigial nuclei.

3. Indicate the other portions of the CNS with which each of the longitudinal zones of the cerebellum is primarily interconnected, and the places (if any) where these connections cross the midline.

4. Describe the contents of the inferior, middle and superior cerebellar peduncles.

5. Distinguish between the effects of damage to the vermis and the hemispheres of the cerebellum. Explain the anatomical bases for these differences, in terms of CNS connections.

The cerebellum helps coordinate movement by sampling most kinds of sensory information, comparing current movements with intended movements, and issuing correcting signals. The comparisons are made in a uniform, precisely organized cerebellar cortex and the correcting signals issued through a set of deep cerebellar nuclei. Since its output is concerned with coordination of movement and not with perception, cerebellar lesions cause incoordination but no sensory changes.

---

1. Mossy fibers and climbing fibers provide the input to cerebellar cortex, Purkinje cells provide the output fibers from the cortex, and deep nuclei provide the final cerebellar output.

Afferents from many places reach the cerebellar cortex as two types of fibers, mossy fibers and climbing fibers. Climbing fibers, all from the contralateral inferior olivary nucleus, end directly on Purkinje cells, which provide the output from cerebellar cortex. Mossy fibers, in contrast, end on the tiny granule cells of the cerebellar cortex; these in turn issue parallel fibers that synapse on Purkinje cells. Mossy fibers provide the nonolivary inputs to the cerebellar cortex. While they arise on both sides of the CNS, the mossy fibers on one side of the cerebellum carry information related to the *ipsilateral* side of the body.

Some Purkinje cell axons project directly to the vestibular nuclei. Except for these, however, the entire Purkinje cell output is directed to a series of deep cerebellar nuclei, which in turn provide the output from the cerebellum.

Fig. 14-1. Cerebellar cortex and deep nuclei

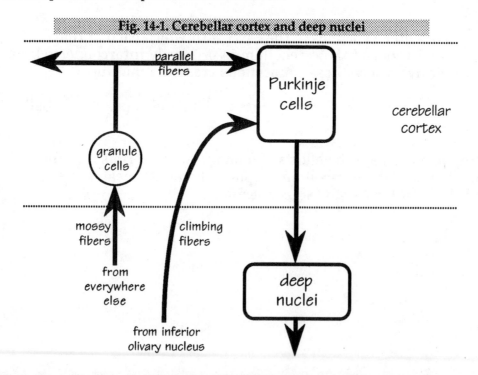

---

2. The cerebellar cortex is divided functionally into three longitudinal zones, each of which projects to a particular deep nucleus.

In a gross anatomical sense, the primary fissure divides the bulk of the cerebellum into anterior and posterior lobes, and another deep fissure separates the flocculus and nodulus (together comprising the flocculonodular lobe) from the bulk of the cerebellum.

In terms of connections and functions, however, it is more useful to divide each half of the cerebellum into three longitudinal zones - a midline vermis, a lateral hemisphere, and an intermediate zone between the two. The vermis is involved in coordination of trunk movements. The intermediate zone and hemisphere are both involved in ipsilateral limb movements, but in different ways. The view in the following cartoons of the cerebellum is as though you were looking from behind (as in text Fig. 14-2, p. 338) at a cerebellum that had been flattened out so that all its parts could be seen.

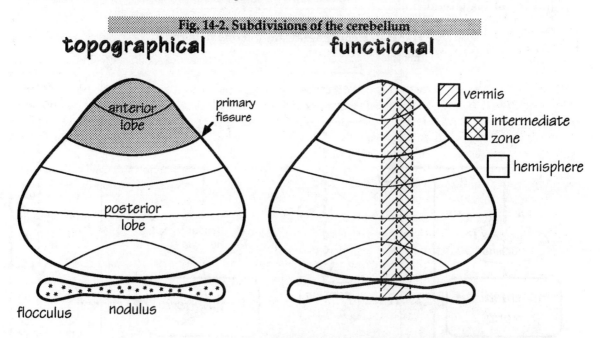

Fig. 14-2. Subdivisions of the cerebellum

topographical

functional

The flocculonodular lobe is primarily concerned with vestibular function (posture and eye movements), and most of its output is directed to the vestibular nuclei either directly or indirectly. The three longitudinal zones of the remainder of the cerebellum direct their outputs to three deep nuclei arranged in a corresponding medial-to-lateral array.

The interposed nucleus is made up of two smaller nuclei (the globose and emboliform nuclei) with similar connections.

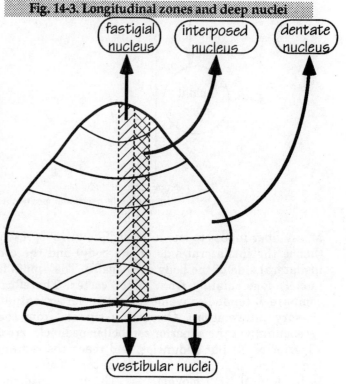

Fig. 14-3. Longitudinal zones and deep nuclei

140

3. Cerebellar inputs and outputs are arranged so that one side of the cerebellum is related to the ipsilateral side of the body.

Each fastigial nucleus, relaying the output from the vermis, projects bilaterally to the reticular formation and vestibular nuclei. However, the intermediate zone/interposed nucleus and hemisphere/dentate nucleus systems of each side are connected so that they help control ipsilateral limbs.

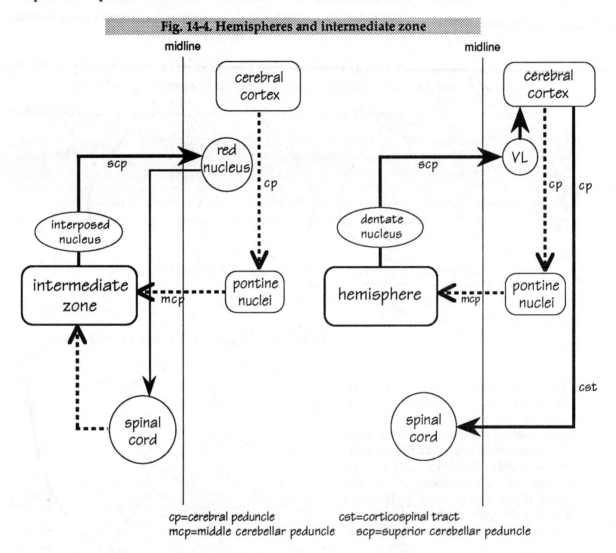

Fig. 14-4. Hemispheres and intermediate zone

cp=cerebral peduncle   cst=corticospinal tract
mcp=middle cerebellar peduncle   scp=superior cerebellar peduncle

Mossy fiber inputs to one intermediate zone represent the ipsilateral half of the spinal cord (hence the ipsilateral side of the body) and the contralateral cerebral cortex (hence the ipsilateral side of the body once again). The inputs from cerebral cortex, by way of pontine nuclei, come mainly from motor cortex. Therefore the intermediate zone is set up to compare intended movement (motor cortex output) and actual movement (spinal cord sensory information). Correcting signals from the interposed nucleus then leave the cerebellum via the superior cerebellar peduncle, cross the midline in the decussation of the superior cerebellar peduncles, and reach the red nucleus. Rubrospinal fibers then *recross* the midline and travel to the spinal cord. Thus the intermediate zone of one side is related to ipsilateral limb movements. (The interposed nucleus can also influence corticospinal output by means of projections through VL of the thalamus; these connections are not indicated in Fig. 14-4, although they are probably more important functionally than the rubrospinal projection.)

Both the inputs and the outputs of the cerebellar hemisphere emphasize the cerebral cortex. Inputs, by way of pontine nuclei, come from contralateral motor, premotor, somatosensory and other cortex. Outputs, by way of the dentate nucleus, the decussation of the superior cerebellar peduncles, and the contralateral VL, return to contralateral motor and premotor cortex. This cerebral cortex→cerebellum→cerebral cortex loop suggests that the cerebellar hemispheres participate in planning rather than monitoring movements.

4. The middle and inferior cerebellar peduncles carry most of the input to the cerebellum; the superior cerebellar peduncle carries most of the output.

The superior cerebellar peduncle is the major output route from its side of the cerebellum, carrying all the efferents from the dentate and interposed nuclei and some of the efferents from the fastigial nucleus. The middle cerebellar peduncle is the input route for information from the cerebral cortex, carrying the fibers from contralateral pontine nuclei. By elimination then, the inferior cerebellar peduncle is a complex bundle, carrying most of the remaining cerebellar afferents (including climbing fibers) as well as the remaining cerebellar efferents.

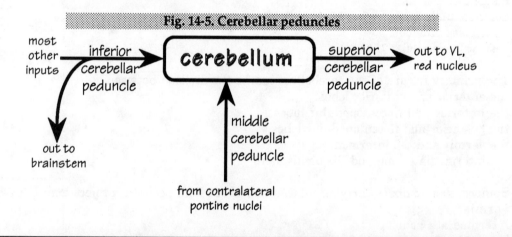

Fig. 14-5. Cerebellar peduncles

5. Cerebellar damage causes coordination deficits, but no sensory changes.

Since cerebellar outputs are directed toward the brainstem and motor areas of the cerebral cortex, cerebellar damage does not cause sensory changes. Rather, such damage causes movement disorders whose nature depends on the part of the cerebellum damaged. If the flocculonodular lobe is out of order, difficulties with equilibrium and with eye movements (especially pursuit movements) result. Damage to the vermis causes incoordination (ataxia) of trunk movements. Damage to the intermediate zone or hemisphere causes ataxia of the ipsilateral limbs.

1. The axons of cerebellar granule cells are
a) parallel fibers.
b) mossy fibers.
c) climbing fibers.
d) the principal output from cerebellar cortex.
e) figments of Jack Nolte's imagination.

2. Most of the output of the cerebellum is in the form of
a) Purkinje cell axons.
b) climbing fibers.
c) axons of neurons in the deep cerebellar nuclei.
d) mossy fibers.

3. The cortex of the cerebellar vermis projects mainly to the
a) fastigial nucleus.
b) dentate nucleus.
c) interposed nucleus.
d) vestibular nuclei.

4. The flocculonodular lobe projects mainly to the
a) fastigial nucleus.
b) dentate nucleus.
c) interposed nucleus.
d) vestibular nuclei.

5. The primary fissure of the cerebellum marks the division between
a) the anterior and posterior lobes.
b) the anterior and flocculonodular lobes.
c) the posterior and flocculonodular lobes.
d) the vermis and the intermediate zone.
e) the intermediate zone and the hemisphere.

6. Spinocerebellar fibers carrying information about limb position project mainly to the
a) vermis.
b) intermediate zone.
c) hemisphere.

7. Information travelling from the right cerebral hemisphere to the cerebellum crosses the midline
a) in the decussation of the superior cerebellar peduncles.
b) on its way from the right thalamus (VA/VL) to the pons.
c) in the pons, as pontocerebellar fibers.
d) This information does not cross the midline.

For questions 8-10, match the fiber types in the column on the left with the cerebellar peduncles in the column on the right; each peduncle may be used more than once or not at all.

8. climbing fibers

    a) inferior cerebellar peduncle

9. output fibers from the interposed nucleus

    b) middle cerebellar peduncle

10 projections from cerebellum to vestibular nuclei

    c) superior cerebellar peduncle

11. There is a small spino-olivary tract from the spinal cord to the inferior olivary nucleus. Based on what you know about cerebellar connections, would you expect this tract to be mostly crossed or mostly uncrossed?

Answers and Explanations

1. **a.** See Fig. 14-1.

2. **c.** Mossy and climbing fibers are cerebellar afferents. Only a few Purkinje axons leave the cerebellum; most project to the deep nuclei.

3. **a.** See Fig. 14-3.

4. **d.** See Fig. 14-3.

5. **a.** See Fig. 14-2.

6. **b.** The vermis and intermediate zone receive most of the spinal afferents to the cerebellum; the vermis is concerned with the trunk, the intermediate zone with the extremities.

7. **c.** This information must cross the midline someplace in order to keep both the left side of the cerebellum and the right cerebral hemisphere related to the left side of the body. The superior cerebellar peduncles are efferent from the cerebellum, and the thalamus does not project to the pons.

8. **a.** Climbing fibers come from the inferior olivary nucleus and make up the bulk of the inferior cerebellar peduncle.

9. **c.** Except for efferents to the vestibular nuclei and reticular formation (which go through the inferior peduncle), almost all cerebellar efferents travel through the superior cerebellar peduncle.

10. **a.**

11. Since olivocerebellar fibers (i.e., climbing fibers) are crossed, spino-olivary fibers would also need to cross the midline in order to keep on side of the cerebellum related to the same side of the body.

CHAPTER 15

CEREBRAL CORTEX

LEARNING OBJECTIVES

1. Name and describe the principal interneurons and principal output neurons of the cerebral cortex. Describe the difference between granular and agranular cortex and indicate which cortical areas typify each.

2. Give two examples of the columnar organization of the cerebral cortex.

3. Describe in general terms the origin and termination of the fibers in the corpus callosum and the anterior commissure.

4. On a schematic drawing of a cerebral hemisphere, indicate the locations of primary motor cortex and primary somatosensory, visual and auditory cortex. Indicate the Brodmann numbers used for each of these areas.

5. On a schematic drawing of a cerebral hemisphere, indicate the locations of the unimodal association areas, i.e., the association areas primarily concerned with motor, somatosensory, visual and auditory functions. Indicate the Brodmann numbers used for each of these areas.

6. On a schematic drawing of a cerebral hemisphere, indicate the locations of the major multimodal association areas, i.e., those association areas in which multiple modalities are integrated.

7. On a schematic drawing of a cerebral hemisphere, indicate the locations of the major limbic areas of cortex.

8. Describe Broca's, Wernicke's and conduction aphasia, and indicate the part (and side) of the brain in which damage causes each.

9. Define apraxia, agnosia and contralateral neglect.

10. Define the term disconnection syndrome and give two examples.

11. Describe the consequences of damage to the hemisphere nondominant for language.

12. Describe the consequences of damage to the frontal lobes anterior to motor and premotor cortex.

13. Compare and contrast slow-wave sleep and REM sleep.

14. Describe in general terms the role of the reticular formation in control of the sleep-wake cycle.

The cerebral cortex is ultimately the part of the CNS that makes us human. Activity of other parts of the CNS like sensory pathways and the reticular activating system is also important, but to a great extent these other parts just serve to let the cortex "do its thing." The cerebral cortex is a big sheet of repeated functional modules, with the operations of the different arrays of modules corresponding to progressively more complex mental functions.

1. Granule cells are the principal interneurons and pyramidal cells are the principal output neurons of the cerebral cortex.

Most areas of cerebral cortex are neocortex, meaning that they have six more or less distinct layers. The two predominant neuronal classes in neocortex are granule cells and pyramidal cells. Granule cells are small multipolar neurons and are the principal interneurons of neocortex. Pyramidal cells are typically larger than granule cells and shaped as their name implies. They have a long apical dendrite ascending toward the cortical surface, a series of basal dendrites, and an axon emerging from the base of the cell body. Most of the axons that leave the cerebral cortex are axons of pyramidal cells.

The four middle layers of neocortex are alternating layers of mostly granule cells and mostly pyramidal cells (text Fig. 15-5, p. 363). Cortical areas that do not emit many long axons, like primary sensory areas, are full of small pyramidal and granule cells and are called granular areas. Cortical areas that emit many long axons, like motor cortex, have many large pyramidal cells and are called agranular areas.

2. The cerebral cortex is arranged in functional columnar units.

Despite the horizontal layering of neocortex, other data indicate that in a functional sense it is organized into columns on the order of 100 μm wide and oriented perpendicular to the cortical surface. Endings in one cortical area from either the thalamus or another cortical area are often organized into such columns, separated by other columns that do not receive such endings. Visual cortex is organized into columns of cells having similar response properties, with adjacent columns differing in one parameter. Likewise, somatosensory cortex is organized into columns of neurons that respond best to a particular kind of stimulus.

3. The corpus callosum and the anterior commissure interconnect the two cerebral hemispheres.

The corpus callosum is a bundle of several hundred million axons that interconnect the two cerebral hemispheres. Many of these fibers project from sites in the frontal, parietal or occipital cortex on one side to the mirror-image sites on the other side. However, others interconnect areas that are functionally related to each other but not mirror images. The frontal and occipital lobes project mostly through the enlarged genu and splenium, respectively, and the parietal lobe mostly through the body of the corpus callosum.

The anterior commissure contains similar fibers that interconnect the temporal lobes; as well as other fibers that interconnect components of the olfactory system.

146

4. Motor cortex is in the frontal lobe, somatosensory cortex in the parietal lobe, auditory cortex in the temporal lobe and visual cortex in the occipital lobe.

Certain areas of cerebral cortex are closely identified with sensory and motor functions and receive the bulk of the projections from the appropriate thalamic relay nuclei. They are therefore called primary areas. Primary motor cortex occupies most of the precentral gyrus, primary somatosensory cortex the postcentral gyrus, primary auditory cortex part of the superior temporal gyrus, and primary visual cortex the cortex in and around the calcarine sulcus. These primary areas contain precise but distorted somatotopic, tonotopic or retinotopic maps with large representations of functionally important areas like the fingers and the fovea.

Several systems have been devised to map the cerebral cortex using various anatomical criteria. The subdivisions in these anatomical maps often correspond to functional subdivisions, and some of the numbers in the map devised by Brodmann are in common use. Important Brodmann's numbers are indicated in parentheses in the following figure and in similar figures in this chapter.

Fig. 15-1. Primary sensory and motor areas

primary areas

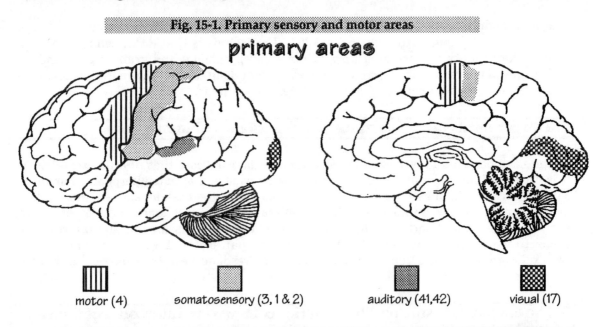

motor (4)   somatosensory (3, 1 & 2)   auditory (41,42)   visual (17)

5. Unimodal association areas are located adjacent to primary functional areas.

Adjacent to each of the primary cortical areas are areas that are involved in the same function and that receive projections from the primary area (and usually from the appropriate thalamic relay nucleus as well). They have less precise somatotopic, tonotopic and retinotopic maps than the primary areas, but their cells have more complex response properties. These are referred to as unimodal (i.e., single-function) association areas. Corresponding to the great importance of vision for primates, there is a particularly large expanse of visual association cortex.

Fig. 15-2. Unimodal association areas

single-function association areas

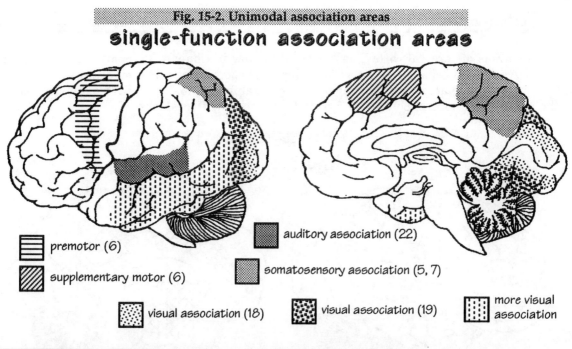

premotor (6)

supplementary motor (6)

auditory association (22)

somatosensory association (5, 7)

visual association (18)

visual association (19)

more visual association

---

6. Complex association areas are located in the frontal lobe and more posteriorly in a parietal-temporal-occipital field.

The single-function association areas send converging outputs to two large expanses of more complex association cortex. The first is a parietal-temporal-occipital region surrounded by sensory areas; it receives thalamic inputs from the pulvinar (which also projects to unimodal sensory association areas). The second is anterior to premotor cortex and is called prefrontal cortex; it receives thalamic inputs from the dorsomedial nucleus. Neurons in these areas may have still more complex properties; they may respond to multiple kinds of stimuli, and may only respond under particular behavioral conditions. Lesions in these multimodal association areas cause correspondingly complex deficits, described in later sections of this chapter.

Fig. 15-3. Complex association areas

complex association areas

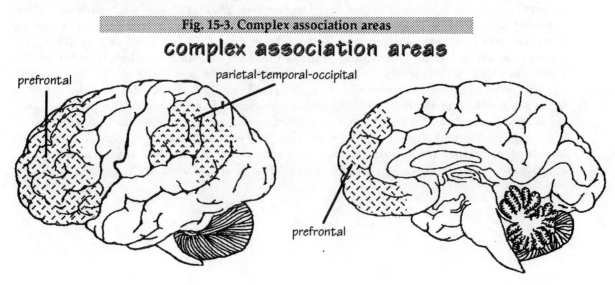

prefrontal

parietal-temporal-occipital

prefrontal

7. Limbic cortex is located in the cingulate and parahippocampal gyri.

Limbic areas of cerebral cortex, as described further in Chapter 16, operate in emotional and drive-related behavior by interconnecting the hypothalamus with other areas of cortex. The major limbic areas are the cingulate and parahippocampal gyri, with extensions onto the insula, the temporal pole and the orbital surface of the frontal lobe.

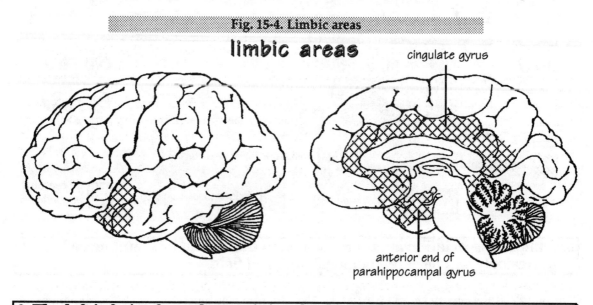

Fig. 15-4. Limbic areas

limbic areas

cingulate gyrus

anterior end of
parahippocampal gyrus

8. The left inferior frontal gyrus is involved in the production of language, the left superior temporal gyrus in its comprehension.

Nearly all right-handed people, and most left-handed people as well, have left hemispheres that are dominant for the production and comprehension of language. Two areas in the left hemisphere are particularly important. The posterior part of the left inferior frontal gyrus, called Broca's area, is involved in the production of both written and spoken language. Damage here causes nonfluent (or motor, or expressive, or Broca's) aphasia in which comprehension is relatively intact but language is produced only with difficulty. The posterior part of the left superior temporal gyrus, called Wernicke's area, is involved in the comprehension of both written and spoken language. Damage here causes fluent (or sensory, or receptive, or Wernicke's) aphasia in which language can be produced but its comprehension is relatively impaired. Affected individuals have difficulty comprehending even their own language, so it is produced fluidly but inaccurately; the result is incorrect words and meaningless phrases. Disruption of the fibers of the arcuate fasciculus that interconnect Broca's area and Wernicke's area causes conduction aphasia, in which an individual speaks and writes like a Wernicke's aphasic, but comprehends language relatively well. Damage to both Broca's and Wernicke's areas causes global aphasia, in which both production and comprehension of language are impaired.

Aphasia	Spontaneous language	Comprehension	Repetition
Broca's	difficult; only essential words produced	relatively OK	poor
Wernicke's	production relatively OK; content defective	poor	poor
conduction	as in Wernicke's	relatively OK	poor
global	poor	poor	poor

9. Complex cortical dysfunction can follow damage outside the language areas.

Damage in association areas of cortex can cause deficits more complex than simple weakness or diminished sensation. Apraxia (from a Greek word meaning lack of action) refers to a condition in which someone is unable to perform a skilled movement in spite of wanting to move and not being weak. Agnosia (from a Greek word meaning lack of knowledge) is a sensory analog of apraxia, and refers to a condition in which someone is unable to recognize objects using a particular sensory modality even though basic sensation using that modality is normal. Neglect syndromes are conditions in which someone is unable to direct attention to one side, and may be totally unaware of one entire side of his or her body. Contralateral neglect most often follows damage to the right parietal lobe.

10. Complex cortical dysfunction can follow functional disconnection of cortical areas from each other.

Normal function of cerebral cortex within the CNS depends not only on the cortex itself, but also on its input and output connections. Hence, disconnection of cortical areas from one another can produce functional deficits similar to those resulting from cortical damage. Conduction aphasia is an example of such a disconnection syndrome, since Broca's and Wernicke's areas are intact but the individual is nevertheless aphasic. There have been cases in which motor cortex was disconnected from language areas, so that an individual was unable to make movements upon request and so appeared to be apraxic. Similarly, disconnection of visual cortex from language areas can render someone unable to read in spite of having otherwise normal vision and language comprehension.

11. The right hemisphere has distinctive nonlinguistic functions.

The left hemisphere of most people is dominant not only for language, but also for mathematical ability and logical, sequential analysis. The right hemisphere, in contrast, is better with spatial and musical patterns and better at solving problems in a more intuitive fashion. The right hemisphere equivalents of Broca's and Wernicke's areas are important for the production and recognition of the rhythmic and musical aspects (prosody) of language that carry much of its emotional meaning.

12. Prefrontal cortex is involved in insight, foresight and social interactions.

Prefrontal cortex receives inputs from sensory and motor association areas as well as limbic areas. It uses these inputs to play a major role in various aspects of personality like initiative, social interaction, insight and foresight. Bilateral prefrontal damage may cause little change in memory or basic intelligence, but can cause emotional lability or flattening, difficulty maintaining attention, diminished drive and curiosity, and decreased creativity. Unilateral prefrontal damage can cause similar but less pronounced changes.

13. During sleep we cycle through dreaming and non-dreaming states, each with distinctive properties.

During wakefulness the electroencephalogram (EEG) typically is either a small, desynchronized signal (during attentiveness) or contains synchronized waves in an 8–13 Hz alpha rhythm (during relaxation). As we fall asleep, the waking desynchronized EEG gives way in stages to a more and more synchronized, slow-wave signal (delta waves, <4 Hz). This state of slow-wave sleep is interrupted periodically by intervals of sleep with a desynchronized EEG like that of wakefulness and bursts of rapid eye movements (REM sleep).

	Slow-Wave Sleep	REM Sleep
Other names	synchronized	paradoxical, desynchronized
EEG	big, slow, synchronized	small, fast, desynchronized
muscle tone	somewhat decreased	almost abolished
arousal threshold	high	higher
mental activity	vague dreams	detailed, complex dreams
ANS activity	slow, regular pulse & respiration; ⇑ peristalsis	irregular pulse & respiration; ⇓ peristalsis; no temperature regulation

14. The Ascending Reticular Activating System plays a central role in sleep-wakefulness cycles.

Sleep is something we do regularly, with a period of about 24 hours. The clock that controls the sleep-wakefulness cycle is in the suprachiasmatic nucleus of the hypothalamus, and its output gets in step with the day-night cycle because of retinal inputs to the suprachiasmatic nucleus. The suprachiasmatic clock then periodically causes the reticular formation of the caudal brainstem to turn off the Ascending Reticular Activating System (ARAS) of the rostral brainstem. This in turn reduces cortical activity and slow-wave sleep is the result.

REM sleep depends on neural machinery located in the caudal brainstem that turns on and off about every 90 minutes during periods of slow-wave sleep.

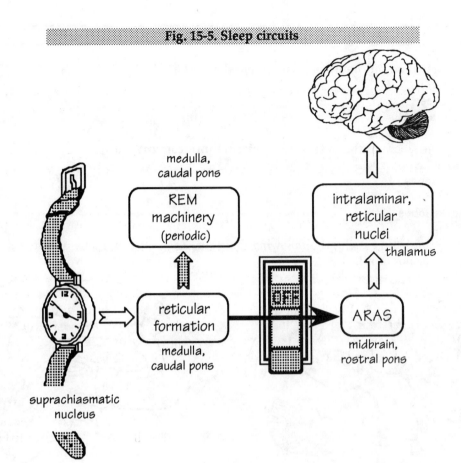

Fig. 15-5. Sleep circuits

1. The principal output neurons of the cerebral cortex are
a) stellate cells.
b) granule cells.
c) pyramidal cells.

2. Most of the fibers in the anterior commissure interconnect the
a) frontal lobes.
b) parietal lobes.
c) occipital lobes.
d) temporal lobes.

Answer questions 3–11 using the following diagram. Each letter may be used once, more than once, or not at all.

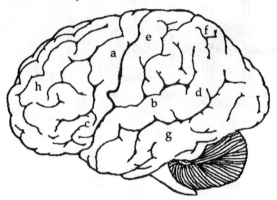 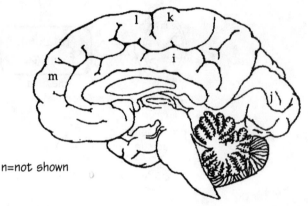

n=not shown

3. Area 17.

4. Agranular cortex.

5. Somatosensory association cortex.

6. Limbic cortex.

7. Supplementary motor area.

8. Area 4.

9. Damage here would cause problems comprehending language.

10. In the right hemisphere, damage here might cause contralateral neglect.

11. In the right hemisphere, damage here might cause speech to be flat and monotonic.

12. REM sleep and slow-wave sleep are similar in that
a) relative to wakefulness, the EEG in both states is of smaller amplitude.
b) both are characterized by detailed visual dreams.
c) muscle tone is almost abolished.
d) the basic neural machinery for both is in the thalamus.
e) none of the above.

Answers and Explanations

1. **c**.

2. **d**.

3. **j**. Primary visual cortex.

4. **a**. Agranular cortex contains many large pyramidal cells with long axons. Primary motor cortex is the premier example.

5. **f**. Parietal lobe, especially the superior part.

6. **i**. The cingulate gyrus which, together with the parahippocampal gyrus, makes up nearly all of the limbic lobe.

7. **l**. See Fig. 15-2.

8. **a**. Primary motor cortex (some at **k** also).

9. **d**. Wernicke's area.

10. **f**. A classic finding after parietal lobe damage, especially the right parietal lobe.

11. **c**. Damage to the nondominant inferior frontal gyrus causes problems generating prosody; damage to the nondominant superior temporal gyrus causes problems comprehending it.

12. **e**. The basic machinery for both kinds of sleep is in the brainstem. The EEG of REM sleep is comparable to the EEG when awake and alert, whereas the EEG during slow-wave sleep is large and slow. **b** and **c** are characteristics of REM sleep.

CHAPTER 16

OLFACTORY AND LIMBIC SYSTEMS

LEARNING OBJECTIVES

1. Describe the pathway by which olfactory information reaches the cerebral cortex, and indicate the cortical areas to which it is distributed.

2. Diagram the general organizational plan of the limbic system as a bridge between neocortex and the autonomic nervous system.

3. Diagram the major circuitry by which the hippocampal formation functions as a part of the limbic system.

4. Diagram the major circuitry by which the amygdala functions as a part of the limbic system.

5. Compare and contrast long-term and short-term memory, and indicate the apparent role of the limbic system in the consolidation of long-term memories.

There is a whole sphere of mental activity that goes beyond simple perception of stimuli and logical formulation of responses. We have drives and urges, and most of our experiences are emotionally colored. This emotional coloring and its relationship with basic drives is the province of the limbic system.

1. Olfactory information reaches the cerebral cortex without passing through the thalamus first.

The olfactory pathway begins with receptor cells whose chemosensitive processes project into the layer of mucus covering the olfactory epithelium. The same receptor cells have thin axons that pass through the ethmoid bone as the olfactory nerve (CN I) and end in the olfactory bulb. Olfactory receptors are therefore highly unusual in having processes exposed to the outside world and in having axons that project directly to the telencephalon. They are also unusual in being neurons that are continuously replaced throughout life.

The olfactory system continues to break the rules by projecting to cerebral cortex without first relaying in the thalamus. The fibers of the olfactory tract, which arises in the olfactory bulb, end in anterior temporal cortex (piriform cortex), as well as in the amygdala and in areas at the base of the brain (anterior perforated substance). Piriform cortex, however, is not neocortex like the cortex that covers most of the cerebral hemispheres; it has a simpler structure and is referred to as paleocortex. There is an additional olfactory area in neocortex, in the orbital cortex of the frontal lobe. In this case the rules are followed: information from piriform cortex reaches the orbital olfactory area via a relay in the dorsomedial nucleus of the thalamus.

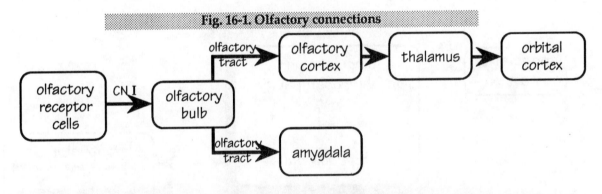

Fig. 16-1. Olfactory connections

2. Limbic structures integrate drive-related inputs and help determine behavioral responses.

We perceive multiple attributes of things—not only their physical attributes, but also whether they are attractive, frightening and so on. Integration of these multiple attributes occurs in the complex association areas of the cerebral cortex (Fig. 15-3), using multiple inputs. Information about physical attributes comes from the single-function association areas, while information about their drive-related attributes comes from limbic structures. Drive-related attributes of objects or situations also have implications for autonomic and behavioral responses, and these are mediated by the same limbic structures in conjunction with the hypothalamus and the adjacent septal area. Hence the general notion of the limbic system is that limbic structures serve as a sort of bridge between neocortex and behavior when drives and emotions are involved (Fig. 16-2).

156

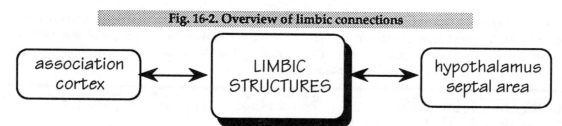

Fig. 16-2. Overview of limbic connections

The limbic structures include both cortical areas and noncortical structures and are divided into two subsystems, one centered around the hippocampus and the other around the amygdala. Each uses different areas of cerebral cortex as part of the bridge to the complex association areas.

3. The hippocampus, together with the cingulate and parahippocampal gyri, interconnects cerebral cortex and the hypothalamus.

The hippocampus (used here to refer to the entire hippocampal formation) is a distinctive area of cerebral cortex folded into the temporal lobe. It is interconnected with the cingulate and parahippocampal gyri, which serve as its bridge to the rest of the cerebral cortex. It is also interconnected with the septal area and hypothalamus (particularly the mammillary bodies) through the fornix, which is the major output route from the hippocampus. The fornix curves around with the lateral ventricle; it separates from the hippocampus near the splenium of the corpus callosum, travels forward in the inferior edge of the septum pellucidum, turns downward in front of the interventricular foramen, and enters the hypothalamus and septal area.

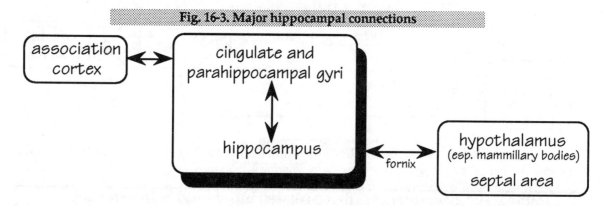

Fig. 16-3. Major hippocampal connections

The mammillary bodies project to the anterior nucleus of the thalamus through the mammillothalamic tract, and this link forms part of a hippocampal loop known as the Papez circuit (hippocampus � mammillary body ➤ anterior nucleus ➤ cingulate and parahippocampal gyri ➤ hippocampus).

4. The amygdala, together with orbital and anterior temporal cortex, interconnects cerebral cortex and the hypothalamus.

The amygdala is a collection of nuclei located in the temporal lobe at the anterior end of the hippocampus. It is interconnected with orbital and anterior temporal cortex, which serve as its bridge to the rest of the cerebral cortex. It is also interconnected with the septal area and the hypothalamus through both the stria terminalis and a more diffuse pathway that travels underneath the lenticular nucleus. The stria terminalis, like the fornix, curves around with the lateral ventricle, but in this case travels just medial to the caudate nucleus; for much of its course it lies in the groove between the caudate nucleus and the thalamus.

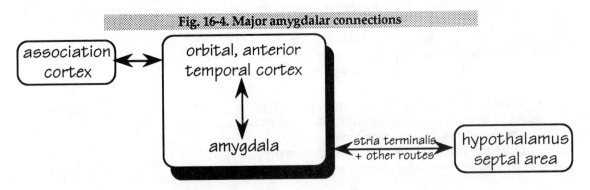

Fig. 16-4. Major amygdalar connections

As implied by the association between the amygdala and orbital prefrontal cortex, the amygdala and the dorsomedial nucleus of the thalamus are interrelated by both direct and indirect connections.

5. Limbic structures are involved in the consolidation of long-term memories.

A simple view of how we learn new facts and concepts is that two qualitatively different processes are involved. The first is short-term memory, a process that depends on directed attention and continuous neuronal activity. Disruption of this process, for example by temporary loss of consciousness, causes loss of all items in short-term memory. Short-term memories are gradually copied, or consolidated, into long-term memory, which probably involves permanent structural and physiological changes in brain synapses. Once something has been copied into long-term memory, it can survive lack of attention and even loss of consciousness and may persist for a lifetime.

Neither short-term nor long-term memories can be localized to a particular site in the brain. Localized cortical damage therefore does not cause inability to form new short-term memories or to retrieve old long-term memories. However, the consolidation process depends upon limbic structures. Bilateral damage to the hippocampus and amygdala causes an inability to form new long-term memories, even though already consolidated memories can still be retrieved; the relative roles of the hippocampus and the amygdala in this process are still being debated, although the hippocampus is generally considered to be the more important of the two. Medial diencephalic damage can cause a similar deficit, presumably because of the importance of the mammillary body and/or the dorsomedial nucleus of the thalamus in limbic circuitry. Acquisition of new skills, as opposed to learning new facts or concepts, does not depend on limbic structures and is unaffected by damage to the hippocampus or amygdala.

Self-Evaluation Questions

1. The majority of fibers in the fornix system connect
   a) the cingulate gyrus to the parahippocampal gyrus.
   b) the hippocampus to the hypothalamus.
   c) the amygdala to the hypothalamus.
   d) the amygdala to the septal nuclei.

2. Bilateral damage to the hippocampus and amygdala causes
   a) inability to retrieve memories from long-term storage.
   b) loss of the ability to learn new motor skills.
   c) inability to "hold" things in short-term memory.
   d) inability to transfer things from short-term to long-term memory.

3. Olfactory inputs reach olfactory cortex (piriform cortex) via
   a) olfactory receptors that synapse on ganglion cells in the olfactory nerve; these ganglion cells project to the olfactory bulb, whose cells in turn project to olfactory cortex.
   b) olfactory receptors whose axons enter the olfactory bulb directly; neurons of the olfactory bulb then project through the olfactory tracts to olfactory cortex.
   c) olfactory receptors that project to the olfactory bulb, which in turn projects to olfactory cortex via a thalamic relay in the anterior geniculate nucleus.
   d) olfactory receptors that are hollow and actually duct the chemical odorants into the olfactory bulb, where a little fan blows them onward toward the cortex.

Use the following list of possible answers for questions 4–8:
a) hippocampus
b) amygdala
c) both
d) neither

4. Is actually an area of cerebral cortex.

5. Receives inputs directly from the olfactory bulb.

6. Projects to the thalamic dorsomedial nucleus.

7. Has a long output bundle that curves around with the lateral ventricle.

8. Interconnected with the septal area.

Answers and Explanations

1. **b.** The fornix is the major hippocampal output route; inputs come mainly from the parahippocampal gyrus.

2. **d.** Short-term memories can still be formed, and pre-existing memories can still be retrieved. Learning of new motor skills is not impaired.

3. **b.** See Fig. 16-1.

4. **a.** The amygdala is a group of nuclei. The hippocampus has a three-layered structure and is sometimes referred to as archicortex.

5. **b.** See Fig. 16-1.

6. **b.** The amygdala uses orbital cortex as part of its bridge to association cortex; the dorsomedial nucleus is connected to orbital prefrontal cortex.

7. **c.** The hippocampus uses the fornix, and the amygdala uses the stria terminalis.

8. **c.** The septal area, together with the hypothalamus, forms the output core by which the limbic system affects behavior and autonomic activity.

CHAPTER 17

CHEMICAL NEUROANATOMY

LEARNING OBJECTIVES

1. Describe the general categories of neurotransmitter molecules, and list the principal members of each category.

2. List the major locations of neurons that use acetylcholine as a transmitter. Describe the location and projection pattern of the major collection of CNS cholinergic neurons.

3. List the major locations of neurons that use dopamine as a transmitter, and indicate which of these neurons have been implicated in Parkinson's disease.

4. List the major locations of neurons that use norepinephrine as a transmitter, and describe their projection pattern.

5. List the major locations of neurons that use serotonin as a transmitter, and describe their projection pattern.

6. Describe the mode of occurrence of peptide transmitters.

161

Neurons typically communicate with one another at chemical synapses, where a presynaptic neuron releases a neurotransmitter, which then diffuses and binds to receptor molecules on a postsynaptic neuron. The duration of action of the neurotransmitter can range from milliseconds to minutes, depending on how rapidly the transmitter diffuses away, is degraded enzymatically, or is taken back up into the presynaptic ending. Many groups of neurons have distinctive chemical "signatures" that allow a different kind of mapping of CNS connections.

1. Most neurotransmitters are either small amines or peptides.

Some neurotransmitters are small amine molecules, and nearly all the rest are peptides of various sizes. The small-molecule transmitters are manufactured in synaptic endings by soluble enzymes and packaged into vesicles there for release. Peptide transmitters are manufactured in the neuronal cell body, packaged into vesicles there, and then shipped down the axon to release sites.

The most prominent small-molecule transmitters are acetylcholine, several monoamines (dopamine, norepinephrine, and serotonin), and two amino acids (glutamate and GABA). Dopamine and norepinephrine are also called catecholamines because each includes the benzene-based catechol molecule (text Fig. 17-4, p. 417).

Fig. 17-1. Important small-molecule neurotransmitters

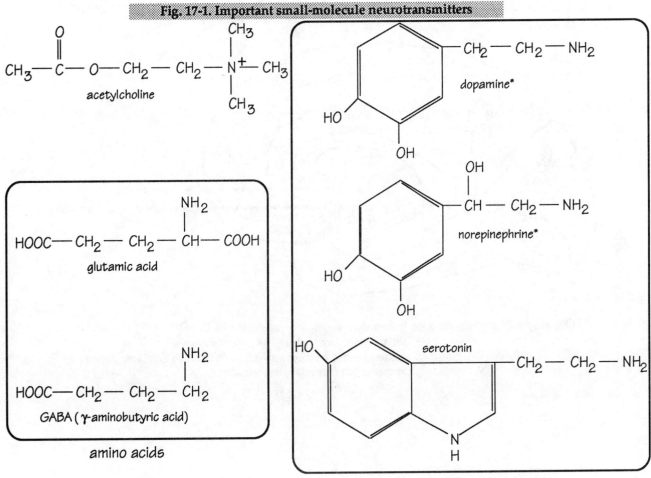

monoamines (*=catecholamines)

2. Cholinergic neurons are prominent in both the peripheral and central nervous systems.

Neurons that use acetylcholine as a transmitter (cholinergic neurons) play an important role in the peripheral nervous system. Some are located entirely in the periphery (postganglionic parasympathetic neurons), while others have their cell bodies in the CNS and axons that travel through spinal or cranial nerves (lower motor neurons, preganglionic sympathetic and parasympathetic neurons).

Some CNS cholinergic neurons are local interneurons in various structures (such as the putamen and caudate nucleus). Others have longer axons that project from one part of the CNS to another. The largest collection of these is in the nucleus basalis (basal nucleus of Meynert), a group of large cholinergic neurons in the basal forebrain (text Fig. A-3, p. 428) that project to widespread areas of the cerebral cortex. Nearby cholinergic neurons in the septal nuclei project to the hippocampal formation. These basal forebrain neurons degenerate in victims of Alzheimer's disease.

Fig. 17-2. Cholinergic neurons

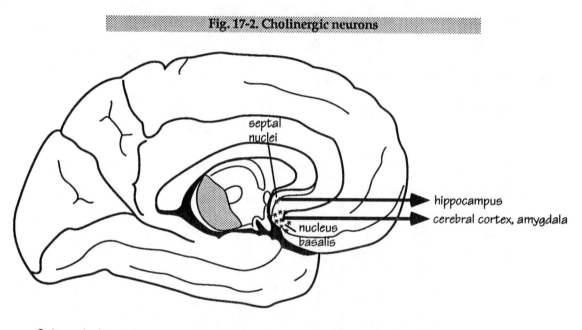

Other cholinergic neurons: lower motor neurons ➠ skeletal muscle
preganglionic autonomics ➠ autonomic ganglia
postganglionic parasympathetics ➠ smooth muscles, glands
interneurons (especially in striatum)

3. Dopaminergic neurons are concentrated in the midbrain.

Most of the neurons that use dopamine as a transmitter (dopaminergic neurons) are located in the midbrain, either in the compact part of the substantia nigra or closer to the midline in the ventral tegmental area. Nigral dopaminergic neurons project to the striatum, and their degeneration has been implicated in Parkinson's disease. Ventral tegmental neurons project to an assortment of limbic structures, and malfunction of these neurons or their targets may play a role in certain forms of mental illness.

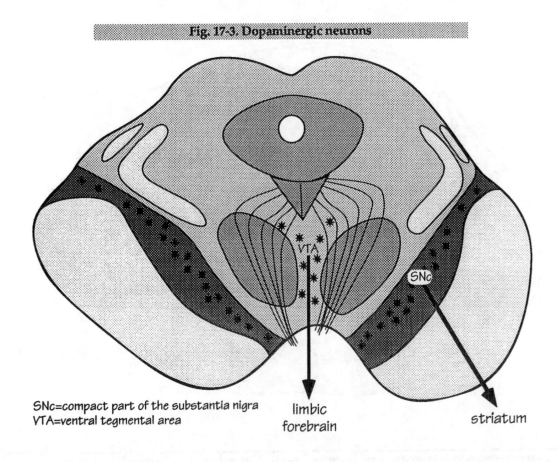

Fig. 17-3. Dopaminergic neurons

SNc=compact part of the substantia nigra
VTA=ventral tegmental area

limbic forebrain

striatum

4. Noradrenergic neurons are located in the pons and medulla.

Neurons that use norepinephrine as a transmitter (noradrenergic neurons) are found in the peripheral nervous system as postganglionic sympathetic neurons. In the CNS, some are located in the medullary reticular formation, but most are pigmented neurons of the locus ceruleus in the rostral pons. CNS noradrenergic neurons collectively project to practically every part of the CNS. The diffuse projections of the central cholinergic, dopaminergic, noradrenergic and serotonergic neurons suggest that all of these play general (but different) roles in adjusting the background level of activity or sensitivity of large parts of the CNS.

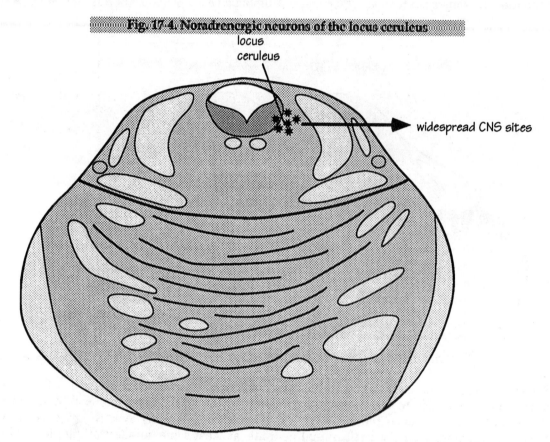

Fig. 17-4. Noradrenergic neurons of the locus ceruleus

locus ceruleus

widespread CNS sites

5. Serotonergic neurons are located near the midline throughout the brainstem.

Neurons that use serotonin as a transmitter (serotonergic neurons) are located primarily in the raphe nuclei, a collective name for a series of nuclei near the midline of the brainstem reticular formation. Like the noradrenergic neurons of the locus ceruleus, the serotonergic neurons of the raphe nuclei project practically everywhere in the CNS, suggesting that they too may be involved in adjusting levels of attention or arousal.

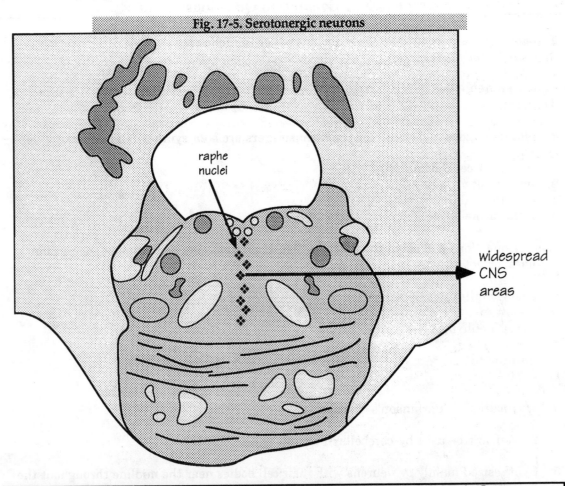

Fig. 17-5. Serotonergic neurons

6. Glutamate is the principal excitatory transmitter, and GABA the principal inhibitory transmitter, in the CNS.

Several amino acids are thought to be transmitters at various CNS sites, but the most important are glutamate and GABA. Glutamate is to the CNS what acetylcholine is to the PNS—that is, glutamate is the mediator of most quick depolarizing synaptic potentials. As such, it is a transmitter for corticospinal neurons, at least some dorsal root ganglion cells, and lots of interneurons. GABA (γ-aminobutyric acid) does just the opposite—it mediates quick hyperpolarizing synaptic potentials. It is the principal inhibitory transmitter, used by cerebellar Purkinje cells and lots of other projection neurons and interneurons.

7. Dozens of different neuroactive peptides function as transmitters.

It was thought for a long time that each neuron synthesized and released only a single neurotransmitter. However, it is now apparent that most or all neurons use not only one of the "conventional" transmitters described above, but also one or more neuropeptides. Many of these neuropeptides had already been known as hormones secreted in other parts of the body, and the discovery that they are also synthesized and released by neurons indicates a previously unsuspected level of coordination between the brain and the rest of the body.

Self-Evaluation Questions

1. Monoamine neurotransmitters include all of the following *except*
    a) acetylcholine.
    b) dopamine.
    c) norepinephrine.
    d) serotonin.

2. Neuropeptides and small-molecule transmitters are *both* synthesized to a great extent
    in
    a) neuronal cell bodies.
    b) presynaptic endings.
    c) both (a) and (b).
    d) None of the above.

Answer questions 3–8 using the following list. Each item may be used once, more than
once, or not at all.

    a) acetylcholine.
    b) dopamine.
    c) norepinephrine.
    d) serotonin.
    e) glutamate.
    f) GABA.

3. Implicated in Parkinson's disease.

4. A transmitter used by cerebellar Purkinje cells.

5. Synthesized mainly by neurons with their cell bodies near the midline throughout the
    brainstem reticular formation.

6. The principal excitatory transmitter in the CNS.

7. Used as a transmitter by neurons of the locus ceruleus.

8. Used as a transmitter by neurons that project from the septal nuclei to the hippocampal
    formation.

Answers and Explanations

1. **a.**

2. **d.** Neuropeptides are synthesized and packaged in the cell body, then shipped down the axon; small-molecule transmitters are synthesized by soluble enzymes in synaptic endings.

3. **b.** Degeneration of the pigmented, dopaminergic neurons of the substantia nigra (compact part) causes Parkinson's disease.

4. **f.** Cerebellar Purkinje cells are all inhibitory, and so use GABA, which is the principal CNS inhibitory transmitter.

5. **d.** See Fig. 17-5.

6. **e.**

7. **c.**

8. **a.** See Fig. 17-2.

168

CHAPTER 18

REVIEW QUESTIONS

The material in this study guide, and the self-evaluation questions that go with the material, has thus far been parceled out into (hopefully) easy-to-digest chunks. This parceling out, however, is only meant to be a stepwise approach to reaching a broader understanding of the overall organization of the central nervous system. This chapter is a series of questions designed to cover all the material in the book. Some of them are simple review questions referring to individual chapters, while others require the integration of material from several chapters.

1. Sensory information arriving at one side of the body or head typically reaches the cerebral cortex of the contralateral side. The axons that cross the midline to accomplish this are the axons of
    a) primary sensory neurons.
    b) second-order or higher-order neurons in the sensory pathway.
    c) thalamic neurons.
    d) Could be any of the above, depending on the sensory pathway.

2. Arachnoid villi are
    a) the sites at which cerebrospinal fluid is secreted.
    b) the sites at which cerebrospinal fluid is filtered out of blood.
    c) the sites at which cerebrospinal fluid is pumped out of subarachnoid space and into the venous circulation.
    d) the sites at which cerebrospinal fluid is pushed passively by hydraulic pressure into the venous system.
    e) small vacation homes for spiders in southern France.

3. Obstruction of the posterior (but not the anterior) part of the superior sagittal sinus can cause increased pressure in subarachnoid space, and has even been reported to cause hydrocephalus. Why?

4. Medial medullary syndrome (the name says something about the location of the lesion) refers to a condition in which a patient has spasticity and diminished proprioception and tactile sensation on one side of the body, combined with weakness and atrophy of the contralateral side of the tongue. Which way would the tongue deviate when protruded? What structures would have been damaged to account for these findings? Occlusion of which artery or arteries would be most likely to cause such a syndrome?

5. A left-handed 65-year-old butterfly collector complains that he has been having more and more difficulty lately collecting butterflies because he "sees double" and gets confused. Your examination reveals a drooping right eyelid, a lateral strabismus of the right eye, and a moderately dilated right pupil. He is completely unable to move his right eye to the left past the midline. You can find absolutely no other neurological disturbances. Following arteriography, the radiologist announces that the patient has a large intracranial aneurysm. You immediately say, "Aha! I knew it! It's an aneurysm of the ..."

6. A 39-year-old handball hustler, in an apoplectic rage over a referee's call, suddenly lost consciousness and fell to the floor. He was rushed to an emergency room and treated for an intracranial hemorrhage. When you examine him several days later, you find weakness of his right arm and leg. Stroking the sole of his right foot causes its big toe to turn up and its others to fan. The patient looks at you with his head turned to the left, because he says that in any other position he sees double. When you ask him to look straight ahead, his left eye is deviated medially. When you ask him to look to the right, his right eye moves normally and his left eye moves further medially. When you ask him to look to the left, his right eye again moves normally, and his left eye moves laterally almost, but not quite, to the midline. The sensory exam is normal and there are no other cranial nerve findings. Where is the damage? Which artery, or a branch of which artery, caused it?

7. A 33-year-old, right-handed roller derby skater comes to you complaining of periodic attacks of tinnitus ("ringing" or "buzzing") in her left ear, and vertigo (the sensation that she and her surroundings are moving relative to one another, when she is standing or sitting still). She says these attacks have been becoming more frequent over the last year or so, and that now, between attacks, she feels as though she can't hear as well with her left ear as she can with her right. Your examination reveals that the auditory threshold is indeed elevated in her left ear. You also notice that touching either cornea with a wisp of cotton causes her right eye to blink briskly and her left eye to blink rather sluggishly. Then you notice that she seems to have a somewhat asymmetrical smile: The right side of her face moves more than the left. What is the most likely cause of this patient's problems?

8. A 57-year-old, right-handed topologist, while discussing the various routes out of Klein bottles, suddenly became dizzy and tumbled to the floor. She did not lose consciousness, but was mildly confused and complained of a severe headache for several days after the fall. Following hospitalization and partial recovery, some symptoms and signs persisted. The patient was referred to you, an eminent neurologist, for diagnosis and treatment two weeks after the episode. Your examination revealed the following:
a) The patient was alert, oriented, intelligent, and showed no sign of confusion.
b) She no longer complained of headache.
c) There was complete loss of pain and temperature sensation on the right side of her body.
d) Her voice seemed hoarse and somewhat abnormal, and her left vocal cord and left soft palate appeared paralyzed.
e) There was loss of pain and temperature sensation on the left side of her face.
f) She complained of often feeling dizzy.
g) Her left arm and leg were mildly ataxic. For example, if she tried to reach for something with her left hand, the hand would oscillate as it approached the object.
h) Her history revealed that she had enjoyed generally excellent health, but had gradually developed hypertension over the previous few years.

Could a single lesion account for all these findings? What structures were damaged? What was the most likely cause?

9. Are there places in the brainstem where a single reasonably discrete lesion could cause:
a) bilateral Babinski signs?
b) bilateral loss of tactile and proprioceptive sensation in the body?
c) bilateral loss of pain and temperature sensation in the body?
d) bilateral signs of cerebellar dysfunction?

170

10. Arrange the following fibers in order of conduction velocity, with the fastest first: afferents from muscle spindles, afferents from temperature receptors, axons of gamma motor neurons.
a) gamma, temperature, spindle.
b) gamma, spindle, temperature.
c) spindle, gamma, temperature.
d) temperature, gamma, spindle.
e) spindle, temperature, gamma.

11. A middle-aged neurologist was walking through City Park late one night wearing a peculiar hat and laughing to himself (as he often did) when he was mistaken for a moose by an overeager bowhunter. The left half of his spinal cord was severed at T12. What neurological problems would you expect him to have a month later?

12. Endolymph
a) fills the bony labyrinth.
b) fills a restricted part of the membranous labyrinth.
c) has a high [K$^+$], relative to ordinary extracellular fluid.
d) none of the above.

13. Deafness of the left ear would be caused by damage to the
a) left cochlear nuclei.
b) right cochlear nuclei.
c) left lateral lemniscus.
d) right lateral lemniscus.
e) Either (a) or (c).
f) Either (a) or (d).

14. The visual field deficits shown below (shaded area=defective) could best be explained by

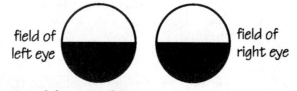

a) Damage in the center of the optic chiasm.
b) Bilateral damage to the temporal lobes.
c) Bilateral damage to the parietal lobes.
d) Damage to the lower half of each occipital lobe.

15. All of the following are specific thalamic relay nuclei *except* the
a) medial geniculate nucleus.
b) ventral lateral nucleus (VL).
c) ventral posteromedial nucleus (VPM).
d) dorsomedial nucleus (DM).
e) anterior nucleus.

16. The anterior limb of the internal capsule contains the
a) efferent fibers from the anterior nucleus.
b) corticospinal tract.
c) corticobulbar tract.
d) efferent fibers from the pulvinar.

Answer questions 17–19 using the following diagram;

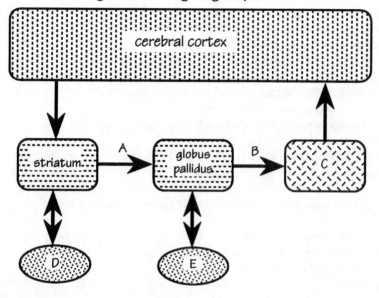

17. Ansa lenticularis.

18. VA/VL.

19. Subthalamic nucleus.

20. Right hemiballismus would result from damage to the
a) right subthalamic nucleus.
b) left subthalamic nucleus.
c) right globus pallidus.
d) left globus pallidus.
e) none of the above.

21. A 37-year-old neuroanatomist and hat designer was involved in a serious collision with a large fish. When you examine him (the neuroanatomist, that is—the fish was unharmed) you notice that when you lightly touch his left cornea only his left eye blinks; when you touch his right cornea, again only his left eye blinks. Which of the following lesions would account for these findings?
a) damage to the right oculomotor nucleus, sparing the trigeminal and facial motor and sensory nuclei.
b) damage in the vicinity of the right abducens nucleus, affecting the internal genu of the facial nerve.
c) damage to the right spinal trigeminal tract, sparing all other systems.
d) damage to the left corticobulbar fibers, sparing the oculomotor nucleus and the trigeminal and facial sensory and motor nuclei.

22. The caudal pons receives some of its blood supply from the
a) vertebral artery.
b) posterior inferior cerebellar artery.
c) anterior inferior cerebellar artery.
d) superior cerebellar artery.
e) posterior cerebral artery.

172

23. Hair cells in a semicircular canal
a) have receptor potentials in opposite directions at the beginning and end of a rotation.
b) continue responding throughout a rotation.
c) are stimulated best by linear acceleration.
d) have sensory "hairs" that are bathed in perilymph.

24. Stimulation of the left frontal eye field would cause
a) slow conjugate movements of both eyes to the left.
b) slow conjugate movements of both eyes to the right.
c) saccadic movement of both eyes to the left.
d) saccadic movement of both eyes to the right.
e) convergence.

25. Increased stretch reflexes in left lower extremity extensors would result from damage to the
a) left cerebellar hemisphere.
b) dopaminergic neurons of the right substantia nigra.
c) right frontal lobe (areas 4 and 6).
d) either (b) or (c).
e) any of the above.

26. Climbing fibers in the left half of the cerebellum originate in the
a) left pontine nuclei.
b) right pontine nuclei.
c) left inferior olivary nucleus.
d) right inferior olivary nucleus.
e) none of the above.

27. The major target of efferents from the putamen is the
a) subthalamic nucleus.
b) caudate nucleus.
c) VA/VL nuclei of the thalamus.
d) globus pallidus.
e) amygdala.

28. The thalamic nucleus most closely associated with parietal-temporal-occipital association cortex is
a) VPL/VPM.
b) the dorsomedial nucleus.
c) the pulvinar.
d) the anterior nucleus.
e) the centromedian nucleus.

29. The embryonic diencephalon gives rise to the
a) putamen.
b) hypothalamus.
c) insula.
d) superior colliculus.
e) amygdala.

30. Real spaces within the cranium include
a) subarachnoid space.
b) subdural space.
c) epidural space.
d) (a) and (b).
e) none of the above.

31. Noncommunicating hydrocephalus would be caused by obstruction of
a) all three apertures of the fourth ventricle.
b) one interventricular foramen.
c) the cerebral aqueduct.
d) any of the above.
e) none of the above.

32. A lipid-insoluble dye injected into a lateral ventricle would do all of the following *except*
a) cross the ependymal lining of the ventricle and diffuse between CNS neurons.
b) move through the ventricular system, out into subarachnoid space, and across arachnoid villi, finally entering venous blood.
c) diffuse across the epithelial lining of the choroid plexus and enter choroidal capillaries.
d) be stopped by tight junctions between the endothelial cells of cerebral capillaries.
e) be stopped by tight junctions between arachnoid cells.

33. A rapidly aging handball hustler, distracted and upset over missing an easy shot during a match with a medical student, ran into a wall at high speed and was unconscious for several minutes. It was later found that he had suffered anoxic damage to the medial part of both temporal lobes. Which of the following do you think was his biggest problem when he went back to playing handball?
a) He couldn't remember the rules.
b) He had forgotten all his trick shots, and couldn't relearn them.
c) He couldn't remember from one day to the next who had won the last game.
d) He had become deaf, and couldn't hear the referee's calls.

34. The dorsal motor nucleus of the vagus sends its axons to
a) parasympathetic ganglia.
b) striated muscle of the pharynx.
c) the solitary nucleus.
d) taste buds in the palate and epiglottis.

35. A 37-year-old goldfish taster comes to your office with a medially deviated right eye, weakness of the entire right side of his face, and inability to move either eye past the midline when he tries to look to the right. A single lesion site that would account for these findings is
a) left frontal cortex, including primary motor cortex and frontal eye fields.
b) right frontal cortex, including primary motor cortex and frontal eye fields.
c) right lateral brainstem at the pontomedullary junction.
d) right medial brainstem in the caudal pons.

36. In both spasticity and parkinsonian rigidity, which of the following is seen in the extensors of the lower extremity?
a) decreased strength
b) increased stretch reflexes
c) increased tone
d) all of the above
e) none of these is seen in both conditions

Use the following list of possible answers for questions 37–39:
a) hippocampus
b) amygdala
c) both
d) neither

37. Efferents through the fornix.

38. Uses the cingulate gyrus as its principal bridge to other cortical areas.

39. Related to the dorsomedial nucleus.

40. Some olfactory tract fibers end here.

1   **b**. Neither primary afferents nor thalamocortical axons typically cross the midline.

2. **d**.

3. Most arachnoid villi protrude into the superior sagittal sinus. Therefore, blockage of the posterior part of the superior sagittal sinus is a form of blockage of CSF circulation.

4   Tongue deviates toward the weak side; damage to pyramidal tract, medial lemniscus and hypoglossal nerve on one side (see text Fig. 9-22, p. 200); anterior spinal or (more likely) vertebral artery.

5. All these findings could be explained by damage to the right third nerve (selective damage to one oculomotor nucleus is very rare). As text Fig. 5-2 (p. 78) shows, an aneurysm at any of several locations near the bifurcation of the basilar artery could be responsible. In fact, the site of origin of the posterior communicating artery is most likely.

6. Weakness of the right arm and leg, with Babinski sign, implies damage to the right lateral corticospinal tract high in the spinal cord, or the left pyramidal tract somewhere rostral to the spinal cord. The eye movement disorder indicates damage to the left abducens nerve and places the lesion on the left side of the caudal pons. See text Fig. 9-5 (p. 183). Damage here, involving a branch of the basilar artery, would account for the findings.

7. The elevated auditory threshold on the left side indicates damage to the left CNVIII or the left cochlear nuclei (but not a more rostral location in the auditory system). Nerve damage seems more likely, since there are no signs of cerebellar damage, even though the the inferior cerebellar peduncle is adjacent to the cochlear nuclei. CN VIII damage would also explain the vertigo. The asymmetrical smile and the sluggish blink reflex indicate damage to the left facial nerve or nucleus. Cranial nerves VII & VIII are close together in the cerebellopontine angle, and the findings can be most easily accounted for by a tumor in this region (e.g., acoustic neuroma).

8. This is a variation on the classic lateral medullary (Wallenberg's) syndrome, caused by a lesion a bit larger than the one shown in text Fig. 9-22 (p. 200). Vertebral or posterior inferior cerebellar artery the most likely culprit. **c** = damage to left spinothalamic tract; **d** = damage to left nucleus ambiguus; **e** = damage to left spinal trigeminal tract; **f** = damage to left vestibular nuclei; **g** = damage to left inferior cerebellar peduncle.

9. **a**, medullary pyramids or pyramidal decussation. **b**, crossing internal arcuate fibers in the medulla, or both medial lemnisci where they are adjacent to the midline in the rostral medulla. **c**, no; the spinothalamic tracts are never near the midline in the brainstem. **d**, decussation of the superior cerebellar peduncles in the caudal midbrain; or conceivably, in the rostral medulla affecting crossing fibers from both inferior olivary nuclei; or crossing fibers in the basis pontis on their way to the middle cerebellar peduncles.

10. **c**. Muscle spindle afferents are large and heavily myelinated, gamma axons medium sized, and fibers from temperature receptors small and thinly myelinated or unmyelinated.

11. Ipsilateral spastic weakness below T12 (corticospinal tract), ipsilateral tactile and proprioceptive deficit below T12 (fasciculus gracilis), and *contralateral* pain and temperature loss beginning a little below T12 (spinothalamic tract). This is called the Brown-Séquard syndrome.

12. **c.** Endolymph fills the entire membranous labyrinth, so **a** and **b** are incorrect.

13. **a.** Afferents from the left cochlea end in the left cochlear nuclei; thereafter, the information is distributed bilaterally.

14. **c.** **a** would cause bitemporal hemianopia; **b** and **d** would cause *superior* homonymous hemianopia.

15. **d.** The dorsomedial nucleus is the association nucleus for prefrontal cortex.

16. **a.** All the others are in the posterior limb or in the retrolenticular or sublenticular part.

17. **b.** The ansa lenticularis and the lenticular fasciculus are the output bundles from the globus pallidus to the thalamus.

18. **c.** VA/VL is the motor relay part of the thalamus.

19. **e.** The subthalamic nucleus has reciprocal connections with the globus pallidus, the substantia nigra with the striatum.

20. **b.** Basal ganglia connections are mostly contained within a cerebral hemisphere.

21. **b.** The right orbicularis oculi, controlled by the right facial nerve, is not working. (Additional deficits would be expected if the MLF or abducens nucleus were damaged.)

22. **c.** **a** and **b** supply the medulla, **d** the rostral pons/caudal midbrain, and **e** the midbrain.

23. **a.** Endolymph keeps moving for a little while at the end of rotation, causing a reversal in the relative direction of flow.

24. **d.** Tracking and convergence are triggered from more posterior regions.

25. **c.** Cerebellar damage often causes decreased reflexes; Parkinson's disease typically is not accompanied by reflex changes.

26. **d.** Climbing fibers originate from the inferior olivary nucleus, cross the midline, and enter the cerebellum through the inferior cerebellar peduncle.

27. **d.** The major basal ganglia circuit is striatum➟globus pallidus➟thalamus➟cerebral cortex➟striatum.

28. **c.**

29. **b.** The putamen, insula and amygdala are telencephalic derivatives.

30. **a.** Subdural and epidural spaces can become actual spaces as a result of certain hemorrhages.

31. **d.** In all of these situations, part of the ventricular system is no longer in communication with subarachnoid space.

32. **c.** The choroid epithelium is part of the CNS barrier system.

33. **c.** Medial temporal damage does not wipe out all old memories or affect skills; auditory cortex is on the superior temporal gyrus.

34. **a.** The major parasympathetic nucleus of the brainstem.

35. **d.** Weakness of the entire right half of the face indicates damage to the right facial nerve or nucleus in the caudal pons. The eye movement syndrome, called a "one and a half" (see text Figs. 9-7 and 9-8, pp. 184 and 185), confirms this.

36. **c.** Neither strength nor reflexes is affected in parkinsonian rigidity. Tone is increased everywhere in rigidity, however, and is selectively increased in upper extremity flexors and lower extremity extensors in upper motor neuron disease.

37. **a.** The amygdala sends its efferents through the stria terminalis and through a ventral pathway under the lenticular nucleus.

38. **a.** The amygdala is more closely related to anterior temporal and orbital prefrontal cortex, although it does have some connections with anterior cingulate cortex.

39. **b.** See answer to (38).

40. **b.** See Fig. 16-1.